Smart for Life

Sasson Moulavi

ISBN 978-1-934209-92-9

Published by World Audience, Inc.

(www.worldaudience.org)

303 Park Avenue South, Suite 1440

New York, NY 10010-3657

Phone (646) 620-7406; Fax (646) 620-7406

info@worldaudience.org

Edited by Kyle David Torke

Dear Readers

The information you'll find in *Smart for Life* is not intended as a substitute for the medical advice and care of your physician; we encourage readers to cooperate with physicians and health professionals in a mutual quest for healthy weight and optimum well-being. *Smart for Life* is not a replacement for individualized medical care, so please consult with a qualified physician and make informed decisions before undertaking any drastic changes in diet or exercise.

Smart for Life has changed the names of individuals discussed in the case studies. We have also provided names for the patients who kindly allowed us to use their before and after pictures.

Dedication

For my wife Renata, my children Eli and Alexa, and my parents Elihue and Shoula—all of whom supported me on my lifelong journey to help improve the health of people around me. Forgive me for not spending more time with you.

"The greatest wealth is health."

—Virgil

Acknowledgments

I have had much help and support during the creation of *Smart For Life.*

First I must thank all the dedicated doctors and medical researchers who paved the way for me because, as they say, when you stand on the shoulders of giants you can see further. I have stood on the shoulders of some of the medical giants who have tackled the worldwide problem of obesity. Many thanks to them for leading the way.

Many thanks also to my research, support, and development team at Smart For Life: Renata, Richard, Tony, Meredith, Elliot, Lisa, Eddy, Wendy (who also designed the book cover), Jimmy, Robert, Maria, Stacy, Anna, Ali, Virginia (who helped me write the book), Gina, Dean, Elvis, Nancy, Shannon, Bruce, Ken, LuAnn, Lorri, Emly, Megan, Sandra, and Sandy.

I also owe thanks to the American Board of Bariatric Medicine and the American Society of Bariatric Physicians, dedicated physicians who have done more with a modest budget than the US government has with the billions spent attempting to combat obesity. The bariatric doctors are down in the trenches every day, working hard to treat people suffering from obesity. Some distinguished members of this fine group include Dr. Mike Steelman, Dr. Allen Rader, Dr. David Bryman, Dana Brittan, MBA, and the ASBP members and lecturers who have shared their knowledge with me.

Thanks to some of our great Smart for Life physicians: Dr. Richard Kowalski, Dr. Allan Magaziner, Dr. Scott Greenberg, Dr. Barry Goldsman, Dr. Larry Klein, Dr. Naveed Shafi, Dr. Michael Kalin, and others past and present. I owe thanks to all the doctors and staff with whom I have worked and trained with: Dr. Guiseppe Dignazio, Debbie from Hawkesbury, Tina, Dr. Danny Samra, Dr. Allen Ben-Hamron ("Ce BON"), Dr. Marc Gagne, the brilliant cardiologist Dr. J.P. Awaida, Dr. Ron Mayer, Dr. Jonathan Bernstein, and Dr. David Klugman among others. I also owe a great debt to the faculty and staff at University of Toronto, McGill University, Toronto General Hospital, Mount Sinai Hospital, Queen Elizabeth Hospital, Royal Victoria Hospital, and Montreal General Hospital where I received my medical training.

My patients at the Smart for Life Weight Management Center in Boca Raton, Florida, have inspired me for many years. Their needs and desires have outlined the map of my research as I looked for an answer to our shared problems with food and weight. I would love to name all of my patients and highlight each of their amazing journeys, but instead I will thank them all here for working with me on this complex puzzle and for honoring me with their trust.

Friends and family have been willing to tell me what they think of my products, and I appreciate the honest input I have received over the years from Juliette, David, Joanne, and everyone from the Unicorn Children's Foundation.

I wish to thank my family for patiently encouraging me to solve my own problem with weight and for accompanying me on the challenging journey from fat young doctor to Smart for Life: Renata, Eli, Alexa, Elihue, Shoula, Gali, Ouri, Joshi, Raphael, Bozena, and Eddy.

Finally, I thank God because with Him nothing is impossible.

Contents

Introduction

Smart for Life has been in the works for almost a decade. As a busy bariatric (that is, weight loss) physician with dozens of weight management centers around the US and Canada, I was asked repeatedly for a book that would explain in detail the Smart for Life weight loss program. I'm a big reader, and I love well-written books on complex subjects. I've wanted to share in book form what I have been sharing with my patients for many years: how to train the body to be healthier and metabolically efficient to get lean, be fit, and slow down the aging process.

I decided I needed to write a book about Smart for Life—but not just any diet book. I wanted to provide readers with comprehensive yet easy to understand information. I wanted not to only share my program but also to reveal the newest science behind eating for health and longevity. I wanted to tell readers the gripping stories of my patients, everyday people like themselves who had suffered from excess weight and obesity, struggled with weight gain and the associated health issues, only to turn their lives around with Smart for Life. I wanted to provide readers with a book they could use on the most practical level, a book with simple menus and delicious recipes. I wanted to give *everyone* who wants to lose weight—whether 10 pounds, 100 pounds, or more—a plan *anyone* can follow safely and successfully.

Smart for Life: Dr. Sass's Solution is the result. Here is my gift to you! But let me explain something: *Smart for Life* is not only the underlying basis for my weight management program. *Smart for Life is how I live.*

I am tall and trim, and I keep myself in good shape. I need to stay thin because of my profession, but I also believe staying fit is the best way to live a long, healthy life. Carrying less weight also keeps us youthful and energetic. I want to live as long as possible and stay healthy and fit for the full length of my very long life. I believe the goal of a healthy, long life is possible. Modern medical science has demonstrated we can, with some smart choices, be healthy and enjoy a long life.

However, there was a time in my life when I was overweight, unhealthy, and generally miserable.

The weight crept up on me. I was never a fat kid. I was a skinny kid and a skinny college student. I was still skinny in medical school. But during the first year of my residency, I began to gain weight.

Residents in medical school work notorious 36-hour shifts, enjoy sleepless days, and eat on-the-run food of questionable nutritional value. At the hospital where I did my residency, the staff constantly ordered food delivered to the staff room from a variety of area restaurants. We all ate when we could from the foods spread out on the large, white tables. The staff room tables seemed always to be lined with food.

For me, breakfast on the go would consist of two donuts wolfed down with copious cups of coffee. Lunch might be half a pizza or a large Styrofoam container of pasta with greasy sauce. Dinner was often Chinese food rich with fried noodles and eggrolls. I paid no attention to the fat or caloric contents of what I was eating. I was busy, and what I ate was the one problem I didn't think about. Besides, I had never worried about my weight. I didn't think I would ever have a weight problem.

Steadily, I gained pounds and inches. My pants grew tight. My normally narrow face became rounder. I didn't really take notice. I kept eating the foods that were killing me.

We all face a similar creep of pounds and fat. Slowly and steadily, insidiously, the weight accumulates. We tend to ignore the extra weight at first, and deny we are getting heavy to ourselves. Eventually, we are forced to face the facts: We are fat, even obese and the extra pounds are affecting our health and our self-esteem.

The extent of my weight gain finally became obvious to me when I was working as an emergency room doctor. In addition to the ER patients, we covered the entire hospital for cardiac arrests. The consequences of my problem were clear whenever I made stat calls to tend to patients whose hearts had stopped beating.

When I received word of a cardiac arrest, I would run up the stairs to the floor where I was needed. Immediately: stat. I always used the stairs to avoid getting stuck in an elevator with patients or hospital visitors who might not understand or could be upset by my need to rush to an emergency. I would jog up four flights of stairs at a pretty fast clip, rush down the hall to the room where I was needed, and start up proper procedures while calling out commands to the attending nurses. I had to be sharp and energetic at all times.

Once I had gained too much weight, I began to notice that by the time I ran up the stairs and rushed down the hall, I was so out of breath and could not talk. I would be huffing and puffing. My distress was embarrassing. I was only in my twenties, not an elderly doctor.

Forced to adapt to my lack of fitness, I discovered to my horror I had to walk more slowly up the stairs to the site of a cardiac arrest. After ascending the stairs, I would walk down the hall to the room where the nurses awaited my instructions. When I arrived, I would not be out of breath, and I would be able to yell commands to the staff. I didn't feel good about how long they had to wait for me. I didn't enjoy other staff running past me and arriving ahead of me.

When I had a moment to myself, in between patients or after an exhausting shift, I would think about how easily I had gained weight. I was at least 40 pounds over the proper weight for my height, yet I had been the right weight only a few years before. I knew I had to do something, but I didn't feel too worried. I figured losing the unwanted weight would be equally as easy.

You probably know what I didn't understand when I was a young doctor: losing the weight I needed to lose would *not* be easy. In fact, I was 100% wrong. As it turns out, the very extent of my misunderstanding about weight loss would form the basis of my current career, driving me to seek answers to the obesity problem and stimulating me to create my own weight loss program. It took me many years to lose the 40 pounds I had so easily gained.

It took Smart for Life to help me lose that weight once and for all, and keep the pounds off. Smart for Life allowed me to safely and effectively attain a healthy weight, one I have maintained now for more than a decade.

If your curiosity is piqued, read on. I'll be sharing the details of my weight loss struggles throughout *Smart for Life*. You will also read about the weight loss journeys of some of my thousands of patients. I have selected more than a dozen of the most inspirational stories to share with you. I want you to be inspired as you read my story and those of my patients. I want you to be reassured: *you can lose weight and keep it off*. There is a way, a healthy way, to lose excess weight once and for all.

But my gift to you comes with a request: I want you to be ON THE PROGRAM while you read. Don't wait until you get to the end of the book to start on the program. Start on Smart for Life right now. I will tell you how.

First you'll need to understand why you are overweight. You need to know why humans as a species are getting so fat. Believe me, you are not the only one who has gained weight. Look around: your family may be overweight. Your neighbors seem to have added girth. Certainly, the people you see downtown or on the bus or in the local movie theatre look a lot fatter than they did when you were young. Have you traveled lately? Some travelers can hardly fit on a plane. They have to reserve two seats. And people in other countries like England, Germany, Australia, and elsewhere are looking much heftier, too. Even the well-to-do Chinese are beginning to suffer from weight problems.

Obviously, we humans are making lifestyle mistakes, and the results are showing up as body fat. But we aren't completely to blame. There are scientific reasons for our increasing problems with weight. The short story I'll explain now. For a longer, more detailed version and all the science behind these facts, you can read Chapter 8: The Smart Body.

Here's what's happening in a nutshell: obesity is a manifestation of a dysfunctional relationship between our genes and our environment. I'm not saying we are destined genetically to be overweight, but there is a genetic component to the problem. *We are genetically programmed to find and conserve energy.*

Energy for the human body is found in food. Our genes are programmed to respond to our food intakes, our food environment. Our genes are receiving messages from our daily food intake, from our diet and its food components, about energy and conservation of energy. Our genes regulate how we process food, and our body's automatic regulatory system has allowed the human race to survive and flourish. The messaging system is how we have survived during long periods of famine. Our genes have been able to protect us against starvation so that we could eat during the good times and squeak by during the lean times.

The gene-food relationship has been an effective system from the start of human civilization. Here's the catch: our diet has changed radically. Most of us no longer hunt for wild meat, pick fresh berries, and spear fish for our meals. The messages our bodies receive from our food environment have also changed. Now, in the modern world, *these messages are the wrong ones.* We are telling our bodies with the food we are eating that winter is on the way and it is time to store up extra fat to make it through the hard times ahead. The problem is that there are no hard times ahead—only more food telling our bodies the same wrong message: store and conserve, turn my food into fat. Therefore, because of the food we are eating, our genes are constantly receiving the message, "it is time to store fat," to convert food energy into fat for later energy needs, with a long winter ahead. After all, our ancestors had to survive. Of course, we don't want to tell our bodies to store fat. Yet, because of the food we eat, we basically force our bodies to convert food to stored fat.

I failed to understand when I was fat and trying to **lose weight** that the modern human diet is creating metabolic dysfunction. Overweight, obesity and all the associated health effects. The overweight body is genetically programmed to store more fat. *The modern diet is turning us into supersized fat-storage machines.*

What I also didn't know back when I had a weight problem was this: To lose weight, we have to change our environment so that our genes can respond properly. Once we alter the environment by changing the food we are eating, we can start sending the right messages to our genes. *We can make our bodies more metabolically efficient.*

The system is complex and involves hormones, insulin, and other complicated body processes. You can read all about it in Chapter 8. All you need to know right now is this: The composition of your daily food intake (environment) is sending signals to your body's cells (genes) that misinform your body about what to do with the energy (food calories) you are consuming. The result is metabolic inefficiency and a body that is really good at storing energy in the form of fat. Which means too much fat in your cells, around your waist, in your face and thighs, in your heart and everywhere else.

The solution to this imbalance is simple, effective, and long-term. When I was overweight, I didn't know what worked, so I spent years doing research until I found out. Then I created a weight loss program based on the research I had done: *We need to change how and what we eat to improve our metabolic efficiency.*

This is exactly what Smart for Life does for you.

There are a number of components to the Smart for Life program that make it unique and successful. You will learn about these as you read this book and follow the program. The main points are these:

1. You will eat six small meals throughout the day and one healthy dinner.

2. You will eat mostly organic, natural, and healthy foods without preservatives or additives.

3. You will eat low glycemic foods to keep your blood sugar level steady.

4. You can choose to include our specially designed food

products to help keep your hunger at bay and improve your overall health.

5. You will not start on an exercise program until you have your metabolism under control. Early on, you'll keep your appetite in check by not exercising until your body is ready. (More on this in Chapter 4: The Smart for Life Exercise Program.)

6. You will make a commitment to the program and we will provide you with support and assistance throughout your weight loss journey.

The Smart for Life diet plan is simple, easy to follow, nutritionally balanced, and delicious. It's convenient, and does not involve a lot of time in the kitchen, weighing foods and cooking. Smart for Life is an on-the-go diet for busy people.

Smart for Life is not a starvation diet. It is not a calorie counting diet either, although it is low enough in food calories to allow for fast and steady weight loss, but not so low that your body burns lean muscle tissue for energy. That's not a healthy or safe way to lose weight.

The Smart for Life diet is well-balanced and appetite satisfying. In fact, we call it a Right Calorie Diet (RCD). Because the RCD is not based on shelf-stable, heavily sweetened, artificially preserved and unhealthy foods. The RCD is natural, organic, and safe.

Most important for weight loss, the Smart for Life RCD does not send the wrong information to your body's cells like other diets do. By eating right on the RCD, you can send positive food messages to your body. That way, you can teach your body to stop storing so much fat. Your metabolic efficiency will return, allowing you to maintain your weight loss permanently. You will also feel and look better, improve your overall health and fitness, and probably change your life.

In fact, by eating less and eating well, you will be sending desirable messages to your body and brain. You will be providing the kind of information your genes require for slowed aging and longevity, as well as improved health and weight control. This means you will probably live longer and feel healthier for many years to come.

That's why *Smart for Life: Dr. Sass's Solution* is the last diet book you'll ever have to read. Once you've corrected your body's metabolism and altered your lifestyle for permanent weight control, you'll be Smart for Life.

Also, you'll cut back on your food expenses. By eating Smart, you won't waste money on unhealthy convenience and fast foods, and you'll get more mileage out of the healthy foods you do eat.

So let's get started.

As another advice to you, I'm cutting to the chase and providing you with the Smart for Life diet, the RCD, in Chapter 1: How I Got Started—and How You Can Too. My advice to you is to *start on the diet program right now, today.* Keep reading this book as you follow the program to learn more about Smart for Life and the science behind the diet, but do get started right away. Obviously, you are motivated right now or you wouldn't be reading *Smart for Life.* Take advantage of your current interest: motivation is essential to success!

In Chapter 1, you'll learn how to select a healthy weight goal and how to begin on the RCD. You'll learn how to destock your pantry. Once you restock with the kinds of foods you'll be eating on the Smart for Life program, you should notice immediately your food bills are significantly lower.

Chapter 2 provides information on appetite suppressants. If you find you are not losing weight on the RCD, there could be an issue with hunger. If you try to follow the diet for two weeks and do not lose weight, perhaps you are too hungry to stick to the program. Battling hunger is not unusual. Don't blame yourself. Around one-fifth of my patients find they struggle against continued hunger cravings. As a result, I have some natural appetite suppressants I can recommend to help with hunger. There are also a couple of prescription medications that work well to suppress appetite. Perhaps medications are blocking your weight loss and/or stimulating your appetite. I will discuss these and related issues in Chapter 2.

On the Smart for Life diet, you won't have to worry about what to eat. I will delineate the spectrum of Smart Foods and Wrong Foods in Chapter 3. I'll tell you about my favorite nutrient-packed Superfoods and the amazing functional foods that help with both weight loss and overall good health. I'll explain why I'm so adamant about including only natural, organic foods in your diet. I'll provide you with Smart meal ideas, shopping tips, and dining out advice.

A vigorous exercise program is not the best way for an overweight person to lose weight. Believe me, I didn't understand exercise wasn't the key to weight loss, and I wasted years of my life attempting to lose weight through grueling exercise regimens. But I *am* an advocate for daily activity. We all should adopt a program of regular daily physical activity and follow the regimen for life. We need to remain active but extreme measures are not necessary, and I'll explain why a time and place exist for eating right and staying active in Chapter 4: The Smart for Life Exercise Program.

Chapter 5: Staying Smart for Life is essential reading. Everyone knows we don't eat solely to satisfy physical hunger. There are many complex psychological reasons for our food choices, and there are social reasons for over-eating behaviors. Some of us sabotage our good eating habits or even have food addictions. In Chapter 5, I'm also going to point the finger at the food industry: they have a major role in your excess weight and the global obesity epidemic now threatening world health. They should be held responsible, and I'll explain why.

In Chapter 6, you'll find menu plans and recipes. Here you'll find the one week menu plan for the RCD. I'm also including a week of menus for the Smart Maintenance program. And I'm providing what I call the Smart for Life Fixed Meal Plan, a stricter version of the RCD. The Fixed Meal Plan works well for dieters who are unable to remain on the Smart for Life diet program because they struggle to avoid temptation. I know how easy straying from the right path and cheating your way off a diet can be. I struggled to stay faithful, too. The Fixed Meal Plan provides a nice kick-start, and most of my patients who try the plan find they are able to switch to the RCD after only two weeks—and stick to the less strict plan. There are more than forty recipes in Chapter 5, including good breakfast foods, healthy lunch and dinner items, delicious snacks, and satisfying beverages.

If you are not interested in all the nutrition and medical science I explored while solving my own weight problem and founding Smart for Life, you can skip Chapters 7 and 8. If you're like me, however, you want to know what the facts are and how food works in your body. In Chapter 7: Get Smart, I share what I learned about diet, disease, and aging, as well as life span. This is exciting stuff! Did you know that eating Smart is good for the health of the planet? You might want to take a look at Chapter 7 and find out why.

In Chapter 8: The Smart Body, you can read the newest science on the complicated systems in your body and brain influencing weight control. Read about genes and body weight; insulin resistance; leptin resistance; nutrients and the effects on blood sugar; insulin and fat storage; hormones and weight; digestion and weight gain (yes, that's right); metabolic efficiency and aging; and other, more complicated aspects of the science of weight control. This chapter is a challenge for those readers who didn't stay awake in biology class, but the research is fascinating. I've included some cutting edge material. Don't let the science intimidate you; you may be surprised at how much you learn.

As a Bonus Section, I'm including important information for parents: the Smart for Life ThinAdventure Healthy Weight Program for Kids. Children face many obstacles when they are overweight. Social ostracism and looksism are issues in today's critical and competitive world. Overweight kids face prejudice from daycare through college and beyond into the workplace. As a young doctor, I was shocked to discover overweight kids are developing what used to be adult diseases at an alarming rate. In fact, today's kids may not live as long as their parents—all because of what they eat.

Fortunately, it's not too late to train your kids to eat smart. ThinAdventure makes eating healthy fun for kids. I'll share the program with you in this Bonus Section of *Smart for Life: Dr. Sass's Solution,* so that you can share the information with your kids.

The Appendix includes a list of suggested books and articles you might want to read plus lots of practical tools for you to use while on the Smart for Life program. Check out the Weight Chart, Food Diary, Exercise Planner, and Menu Planner. You can reproduce these or tear them out of the book for handy use. There is also a website code and access to Live Chat with Dr. Sass, so that you can come to the Smart for Life website whenever you want to get the support you need while you are on the program. Product information guidelines will help you to find what you need while you are becoming Smart for Life.

Ready to get started? Good. That's the spirit. Before you begin on the Smart for Life program, please take a minute to read the following story about one of my most successful patients. She's an inspiration to me and may prove to be one to you, too.

Marnie F.

Marnie F. is a svelte, fashionable woman who lives in upscale Boca Raton, Florida. People meeting her for the first time have no idea she once weighed more than 350 pounds.

Over the years, Marnie had gained way too much weight. She was unhealthy and felt unattractive. She had developed asthma, her circulation was poor, and she was on a variety of medications for disorders related to her ballooning weight.

One day a close friend told her about Smart for Life. Marnie's friend was enjoying success on the weight loss plan and talked it up. Marnie was intrigued, and something clicked inside her mind: she simply decided to change her life once and for all. And the changes worked.

Marnie set a weight loss goal of 212 pounds. Two hundred pounds is an enormous amount of weight. But Marnie was in no hurry.

She wanted to lose the pounds in a healthy manner and learn to eat differently so she would never regain the weight.

She adapted to the Smart for Life diet easily. She learned how to control her hunger and cravings for unhealthy foods. The Smart for Life program provided her with the information and support she needed to change the way she ate and ultimately the way she lived.

It took more than 2 years, but Marnie eventually reached her goal: after adjusting her eating habits and staying with the program, she weighed 138 pounds. Now, 6 years later, she remains at this healthy weight. And she feels—and looks—like a whole new woman. "Everyone tells me that the person they knew before and the person they see today are two different people," she says.

Marnie began to dress differently, developing a striking fashion sense and a style of her own. "My kids always tell me I'm beautiful. The way people look at me has changed. I have more confidence."

Marnie's health improved dramatically. She was able to discontinue her asthma medication, and she no longer suffers from symptoms. She doesn't need to take any medication for her circulation either. "I'm not bloated anymore," she says. "I am very healthy. My kids don't worry anymore about my health."

When asked for her diet maintenance tips, Marnie F. suggests the following: "When it comes to parties, I don't eat. I just drink a glass of champagne. On holidays, I try to eat as healthfully as I can. And whenever I'm socializing, I don't eat anything. I join in by drinking a glass of wine or champagne."

Not such a painful plan, right?

Read on, and you'll soon be Smart for Life, too.

Part I: How to Become Smart for Life

"If I am not for myself, who will be for me?"

—Hillel

"Obstacles are those frightening things you see when you take your eyes off your goal."

—Henry Ford

Chapter 1: How I Got Smart—and How You Can Too

Anyone can be Smart for Life. I'm going to show you how. After reading this chapter, you'll be on your way, and you'll see just how simple being smart is.

But I must admit, I wasn't always so smart myself. In fact, when I was a young doctor, I only *thought* I was smart. Then one night I realized that, despite my education and training, my quick mind and medical degrees, I was ignorant about my own health. Dangerously ignorant.

The emergency room where I worked was located at an inner city hospital in an urban center. We treated a wide array of ethnic groups living in the area. I treated a diverse cross-section of people with different cultures, diets, and languages. The ER was in a section of the city known as "Little Italy." I enjoyed the people I met—and the area restaurants.

One night, I was on duty when a young family man was rushed in by ambulance. He was in full cardiac arrest. The guy was 36 years old, quite a few years older than I but young enough that I felt a connection to him. He was dressed in a nice suit and an expensive tie. He had been out to dinner with his family when he suddenly keeled over.

I immediately began emergency procedures. He was already blue, his skin reflecting the lack of circulating oxygen. He wasn't breathing. I intubated him using a long tube to clear the airway and provide him with oxygen. He vomited a large volume of what looked like spaghetti in red sauce. I was dressed in hospital greens, which I wore constantly at the time because the elastic waist allowed for comfort. Tight pants do not feel comfortable when you are as overweight as I had become. My greens were splattered with pasta and tomato.

Although I tried my best to revive the man, after 45 minutes it became obvious he was too far gone. I stood in the resuscitation room, covered with the man's vomit, trying to accept the fact there was nothing I could do. A young man was dying, and his family waited beyond the double doors for me to exit and tell them his fate. The situation made me feel helpless and sad.

The wife was petite with big brown eyes. She was young, maybe 30. The kids were small, a couple of babies and a toddler. They were surrounded by a big network of relatives, at least 20 family members who had gathered to offer their support. Everyone was speaking Italian. The guy's parents were there, too, sitting beside the dying man's wife. I appreciated how the Italians always seemed to come together in an emergency, providing necessary support to loved ones.

I needed to ask the family for some information. Despite her shock, the wife was willing to discuss her husband with me. "He has no medical problems," she told me. "My husband has always been healthy." At the restaurant that evening, he had complained of chest pains during dinner. Then he collapsed, tumbling from his chair onto the floor. One minute he was joking and eating pasta with his family; the next minute he was lying on the restaurant floor, unconscious.

I returned to the resuscitation room where my team worked on the Italian fellow, trying desperately to save his life. But we were unable to revive him. There was nothing we could do. The man was dead.

My job as an emergency room doctor included informing the family when a patient did not make it. Informing family members about a death is inarguably the worst part of any doctor's job. Notifications are especially difficult when the deceased is young and healthy, the death a sudden shock. I couldn't understand why this man had suffered a fatal heart attack at age 36. Except for his weight, the guy seemed perfectly normal. Except for the fact that he was around 30 or 40 pounds overweight. About as overweight as I was.

When I returned to the ER waiting room, a small crowd of friends and family surrounded the widow. I had to announce to them their loved one had passed. When somebody asked why, what had been the cause of death, I said, "I don't know. But given the fact that he had chest pains and was significantly overweight, it was probably a heart attack." The widow was devastated. There wasn't a dry eye in the room.

A few days later, the autopsy report confirmed my suspicions. The young man had suffered a massive heart attack due to severely blocked coronary arteries. His faulty diet and excess weight had caused his premature death, of that I was certain.

What a waste, I thought. And then I began to consider my own faulty diet and my own excess weight. What did my coronary arteries look like? I wondered. Even though my blood cholesterol was in the normal range, I certainly didn't feel as healthy as I once had. The Italian guy was only 36. How long would it take me to arrive at an ER with a blue face and a set of clogged arteries?

That was the first time I realized how important it was for me to do something about my weight.

Years later, I would attain and maintain a healthy weight. Before I became Smart for Life, however, I would try and fail many times during what became a personal crusade for me: the search for a method to achieve successful, permanent weight loss. You will read more about my attempts in future chapters. Right now, I will give you the information it took me so long to discover: how to eat so that your body stops storing too much fat.

Medical Waiver

Before you go on any weight loss regimen, it's imperative to have either your doctor's approval or medical supervision. If you visit a Smart for Life Weight Management Center, your diet will be medically supervised by a properly trained physician and staff. If you decide to go on the Smart for Life program at home while reading this book, it is a good idea to check with your doctor first. You'll be able to tell him or her all about the diet after you finish reading this chapter. Or you can make an appointment and take the book with you.

Doctors tend to approve of the Smart for Life diet. The program is scientifically and medically sound, nutritionally balanced, and good for your overall health. The truth is, doctors rely on Smart for Life to lose weight themselves. My patients sometimes tell me they see their own doctors in the waiting room at the Smart for Life Weight Management Centers here in South Florida. I'm not the only physician who has to control his weight.

Most doctors know how important it is for their patients (and themselves) to maintain a healthy weight. I've provided a lot more information on the link between diet and disease in Chapter 7, but let me just summarize here—just in case you need more reasons to begin on the Smart for Life program.

Obesity is either the root cause of or a contributing factor in a number of medical diagnoses including heart disease, hypertension (high blood pressure), stroke, metabolic syndrome, insulin resistance, diabetes, arthritis and orthopedic problems, asthma, sleep apnea, cancer, hormonal imbalances, gallstones and intestinal disorders, neurological problems, possibly Alzheimer's disease, and poor immune system function.

All these conditions may be avoided, improved, even eradicated by attaining and maintaining a healthy weight.

Obesity reduces your longevity, too. But if you're fat and sick all the time, living longer may not sound so great. Longevity is associated with appropriate body weight. And living longer goes hand in hand with feeling good, looking good, and loving your life.

SASSON Technology and You

You might think it's funny that I named the weight loss technology I created after myself, but I did so because the acronym makes the system easy to remember. SASSON Technology for weight loss and the food products that form the basis of the diet itself are based on this scientific doctrine: *to lose weight safely and permanently while achieving a state of improved health, the body will need Smart Appetite Suppressing Sustained Organic Nutrition.* This is SASSON Technology.

So what does such a fancy phrase translate to on a practical level? What does SASSON Technology mean for you right now? It means eating a series of small, healthy meals throughout the day. The foods you eat should be appetite suppressing, not appetite stimulating. Your daily diet should contain as much organic food as you can buy—foods in their natural state, minimally processed foods without additives and preservatives. Your daily diet should satisfy your nutritional needs as well as your appetite.

And you should have enough good food to eat so you do not feel like going off the Smart for Life diet. This is key: you'll need to eat regularly, eat well, and stick to the program as the SASSON system becomes a way of life for you.

When patients first come to see me at a Smart for Life Weight Management Center, I examine them and test them to make sure they have no underlying medical issues that need to be addressed. Then I explain to them the basics of the Smart for Life program. I tell them about SASSON Technology and give them the Right Calorie Diet

(RCD), our Smart for Life diet plan, which you can read about in the pages that follow.

My patients usually purchase some of the various products I have developed to help them follow the program. Smart for Life products are based on SASSON Technology and include specially formulated cookies, protein bars, muffins, shakes, soups, beverages, and other items. You can read all about Smart for Life products on our website where you can order these foods in various quantities.

However, you do not *have* to use Smart for Life cookies and other meal replacement products if you don't want to buy them. The Smart for Life diet plan does not require you eat only our prepared foods. My patients usually do choose to use the Smart for Life products, however, because they tend to be busy people who don't want to take the time to prepare special meals and snacks for themselves. You know yourself best, and, once you read over the diet plan that follows, you can make the best choice for yourself and your lifestyle.

Not to force the issue, but I must say I'm pretty proud of Smart for Life foods and beverages. They are 60% organic and contain only the best ingredients, including triple filtered water that is as pure as you can get. No preservatives or other unhealthy additives are included. We use no artificial food dyes or anything like them. Listen: I eat my own products every day, so I make sure they are tasty, healthy, and really good for you. I'm not going to advise you to eat anything I wouldn't eat myself.

Your BMI and Healthy Weight Goal

Before you start on your weight loss journey, you need to know where you're headed. Where are you now, and where do you want to end up?

When a patient is ready to begin on the Smart for Life program, we plan out their journey together. First we measure the patient's body mass index or BMI when she or he weighs in. That's the starting point of the journey, the Before. Then I help my patient to select a healthy weight goal: the After.

The BMI is a weight-for-height index used by physicians for their patients. The BMI chart below illustrates the standard measurements of a weight to height ratio that is normal, overweight, or obese. Your BMI can be used as an indication of the percentage of your body weight that is stored fat: a high BMI means more fat (versus muscle and bone) in your body while a low BMI indicates a lower percentage of body fat.

Studies show that individuals who have a BMI in the normal range have a better life expectancy and lower rates of chronic diseases, including diabetes and heart disease.

Before you decide you're aiming for a BMI of 0, let's review some basic anatomy. A certain percentage of body fat is essential to health and wellness. Body fat cushions your joints, protects body organs, and helps to regulate body temperature. Essential nutrients known as fat-soluble vitamins are stored in your body fat. So it is unwise to reduce body fat too much. A little body fat is essential to good health.

Plus, a little body fat helps to smooth out our muscles and skin. Ever notice how people who are too thin may appear more wrinkled and aged than heavier people? The right amount of body fat helps you look better. Also, long-term studies show that people with a very low BMI have a lower life expectancy. So it is smart to aim for a BMI in the normal range.

Smart for Life® BMI Chart

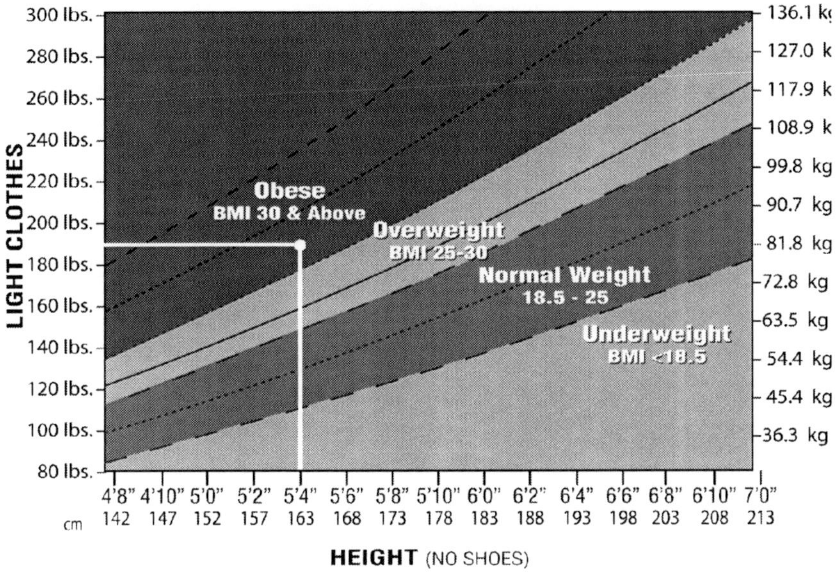

How to calculate your BMI:
Find your height. Draw a line up to your weight and see where you fall.
Example: 5'4" 190 lbs. falls into obese category.

The range for a normal amount of body fat depends on your age. As we get older, the normal range changes, shifting higher. Older people tend to have less muscle, less bone, and more fat per pound of body weight. A normal amount of body fat for someone in their 50s or 60s is greater than the normal level for someone in their 20s or 30s. So older people can have a bit more body fat than younger folks and still be healthy.

Use the BMI charts to determine a healthy weight goal for yourself. You know what you'd like to weigh. Some people select a weight goal roughly equivalent to what they weighed in high school or whatever they weighed when they got married. Others select a weight goal based on how much weight they wish to lose, like 30, 40 or 50 pounds less than whatever you weigh today.

That reminds me: what *do* you weigh today? I know admitting your weight is painful, but you need to face up to the facts about your current weight. So you might as well find out what your current weight is. If you were one of my patients, I'd ask you to step on the scale. Right now. With light clothing on. No heavy sweaters or jackets but no need to stand on the scale naked, either. Do remove your shoes.

Don't delay. Just do it. Go get on a scale. And as you look at your current weight, tell yourself this: *This is the last time I will weigh this much. Ever!*

Record today's date and your weight on the Weight Chart form given in Appendix B: Before. Then record your weight goal. This will be your After.

Sensible Weight Loss

Now that you are about to start on the Smart for Life program, let's talk about how much weight you can expect to lose every week because I want you to weigh yourself once a week and record your weight each time on the Weight Chart in the Appendix. That way, you can track your progress.

Next week, once you have followed the RCD for 7 full days, weigh yourself and record your new weight. Repeat this process every week until you reach your goal weight.

Please: do yourself a big favor and be realistic. Don't expect to lose 30 pounds the first week. Drastic weight loss is not possible, nor is it desirable. You took years to pack on the excess weight, so it will take some time to lose it all. And you want to lose body fat, not muscle and bone. Right?

At the Smart for Life Weight Management Centers, we see patients lose an average of 10 to 15 pounds a month. Some lose more than that, others less. But on average, we see a loss of 2 to 4 pounds a week, which could mean a loss of 24 to 48 pounds in only 3 months. Or a loss of 100 or more pounds of fat in a year.

This is incredible weight loss, and this is sensible weight loss.

This is the kind of sustained weight loss that gets you from the beginning of your journey to your goal. This is the kind of sustained and satisfying weight loss that helped one of my patients achieve amazing success. Here's her story.

Bethany M.

When Bethany M. saw the photos of her sister's wedding, she was shocked and disgusted with herself. She looked huge. There was no denying her girth anymore. It was time to do something about her weight. "I saw myself in the pictures, and I couldn't believe how overweight I was," she says. "I guess I never truly saw myself as heavy as I actually was."

At the time, Bethany weighed more than 340 pounds. She began a serious work out program and totally changed her eating habits. It took a long time, but with months of hard work, she eventually lost 100 pounds.

Suddenly, Bethany stopped losing weight. She continued to eat a balanced diet and work out with weights, but her own weight had plateaued. As time passed with no weight loss, Bethany became more and more discouraged. Was she destined to a lifetime of being fatter than she wanted to be?

"Then a client of mine told me about the diet she was on. I was skeptical at first, but after watching her drop the pounds, I decided to give it a try."

The diet was Smart for Life.

When Bethany started on the Smart for Life program, she was only halfway to her goal. She needed a diet plan that would help her lose another 100 pounds. The diet had to be one she could follow easily, one that would give her the energy she needed to keep working out. She had fallen in love with weight training. Exercise had become an important part of her life.

To her surprise, Bethany immediately liked how she felt on Smart for Life. And she began to lose weight again. She was able to follow the program and not feel hungry. Bethany quickly learned how to eat several small meals throughout the day and how to prepare a healthy dinner at night. She remained on the program, and the weight steadily melted away.

Bethany eventually reached her weight loss goal. After a year on the program, she had lost a total of 105 pounds!

That was more than four years ago. Bethany is now a professional bodybuilder who enters figure competitions. "I placed fifth in my category in the last show," she reported recently. "I do not really struggle anymore with my weight. I have come to trust my knowledge of weight loss and to trust myself. Through eating for competitions and Smart for Life, I have learned so much about how my body works." In fact, Bethany developed an interest in nutrition and is now completing a bachelor's degree program in that field.

Bethany M. looks incredible, and she feels good. She now uses the Smart for Life diet plan whenever she needs to fine-tune her body size for an upcoming competition. She says, "I feel comfortable maintaining my weight, and I know when to turn to Smart for Life for encouragement."

The Right Calorie Diet

The Smart for Life diet program begins with the Right Calorie Diet or RCD. The RCD has been formulated and reformulated over the years, designed and redesigned to insure safety and success. The RCD allows you to lose pounds and inches quickly and permanently. And, after following the RCD diet to achieve your weight goal, you will have trained your body to be metabolically efficient.

The RCD provides you with a reduced caloric intake using healthy foods for proper nutrition, leading to steady weight loss without hunger. Meals and snacks are specially balanced to send the right messages to your body's cells, reeducating your body on proper caloric usage and body fat storage.

Menu plans and recipes for the RCD are provided in Chapter 6. In the meantime, here are the basic facts you need to understand the diet plan.

1. You will eat six small meals throughout the day and one healthy dinner.

Many overweight people do not eat during the day. In fact, most of my patients tell me that they skip breakfast. I will share with you what I tell them: skipping meals turns your body into a fat storage machine. Starving yourself all day, bulking up at dinner and during the evening hours, is the worst thing you can do to lose weight. *By skipping meals, you are teaching your body to be metabolically inefficient.* Your body will adapt to starvation mode during the day and then store the food calories when you do eat. Bottom line: all those late-day and night overindulgences are adding to your fat stores.

A Little History

Smart for Life meal replacement "cookies" are not really cookies. They don't look like vanilla wafers and don't taste like ginger snaps. They are well-balanced mini-meals that provide milk protein, egg white, soy protein, whole oats and other complex carbohydrates, healthy fibers, and heart healthy canola oil. Some of our products contain flax seed, fish oil, and special fibers. All of these nutritious food ingredients help you to stay healthy while you lose weight.

You should be aware of the fact that the human digestive tract hasnot changed much since primitive times. Our ancient ancestors consumed many small meals throughout the day in order to obtain the energy they needed to hunt and gather and to stay alive. Primitive peoples grabbed some berries for breakfast, speared a fish for lunch, nibbled on grains in the afternoon, and then cooked a small animal at dusk. It is only in modern times that we began dividing our food intake into three meals. The results have not been good for us.

Unlike our ancestors, we have become unhealthy, overweight and obese, because our bodies were not designed to eat the way we do now. We need to eat like our ancestors did, dividing our food into small meals throughout the day. Our bodies still need lean proteins, whole grains, lots of fiber, and healthy fats—the kind of foods included on Smart for Life, and the kind of ingredients in the Smart for Life meal replacements.

Some of my patients tell me they cannot control their eating at work or when they are home all day, alone, or with small children. Holidays, parties, and food available on the job all can contribute to unplanned over-eating. This is why I teach my patients to *be prepared.* Once my patients begin on the RCD plan, they know what to eat and do so happily. You too will follow the RCD, eating six small meals and one healthy dinner each day. You won't be hungry and can therefore avoid unconscious snacking, overindulging at day's end, and midnight munchies.

So, what will you be eating on the RCD? Plenty of fresh produce, lean protein foods, and salads. Each day, you will eat a Smart breakfast and lunch plus four Smart snacks. Each night, you will have a healthy dinner. Your Smart dinner will consist of 10 to 12 ounces of lean protein and five servings of veggies.

2. You will eat organic, natural, and healthy foods without preservatives or additives.

If you eat like most Americans, you are consuming far too much convenience food, fast food, and the shelf-stable food astronauts use in outer space. These modern creations euphemistically called "foods" are loaded with salt, sugar, and other preservatives with chemical names as long as your little finger. These foods are not health-enhancing. They may be quick and easy, but the choice and concentration of ingredients are unbalanced nutritionally with excesses of unhealthy fats, cholesterol, sweeteners, sodium, artificial colors and flavors, and other questionable additives. Current research investigating the links between the ingredients in commercially prepared foods and various chronic diseases is, in my mind, striking. If we want to be lean, healthy, and long-lived, we should avoid overly processed foods.

Following the RCD will teach you how to eat healthy foods that fill you up while providing the nutrients your body requires. The RCD diet plan results in just the right balance of healthy foods and nutrients.

As you lose weight, you will become adept at avoiding commercially prepared and over-processed foods. You will eliminate from your life the unnatural foods you no longer wish to put in your body. The RCD teaches you to enjoy eating healthy, the kind of diet you can live on—for a lifetime.

3. You will eat low glycemic foods to keep your blood sugar level steady.

The way the body's blood sugar responds to different foods is known as the "glycemic index." The glycemic index is a reasonably accurate measure of how your body's insulin will respond to the intake of specific foods. The higher the glycemic index, the greater the blood sugar and insulin response. By minimizing the glycemic index of our food intake, we can minimize the insulin we are secreting.

Why does this matter? Well, the truth is, the foods that have the greatest effect on our blood sugar and insulin levels are the foods that result in the most fat storage. Medical scientists and nutritionists have known for years which foods are the most fattening: concentrated sources of carbohydrates. These are the foods that we digest most quickly and find ourselves hungry again soon after eating. Plus, high glycemic index foods flood the bloodstream with sugar (or "glucose"). Our blood sugar levels rise quickly, insulin rises in response, and our fat cells store all the glucose as fat. More on this in Chapter 8.

The RCD is a low glycemic index diet. All the foods you will be eating have minimal impact on your blood glucose, insulin secretion, and fat storage. This is how Smart for Life works. Plus, you won't feel hungry soon after eating. Remember SASSON Technology? The third "S" is for *Sustained.* Eating low glycemic foods allows for a sustained release of energy from your food, and a slower release prevents the sharp peaks and valleys in blood sugar that cause hunger pangs.

Many of my patients are diabetic or have insulin resistance. More on insulin in Chapter 7, but the short story is this: a diet of low glycemic foods can help minimize blood sugar levels to control and even reverse diabetic symptoms. After losing weight on the Smart for Life program, patients with type 2 diabetes often find they no longer need medication.

Eating a diet full of high glycemic foods has become the norm and is, in my opinion, the root cause of the frightening increase in type 2 diabetes in the world population. We can reverse the trend simply by eating less processed foods and avoiding added sugars like sucrose, fructose, corn sweeteners, high fructose corn syrup, dextrose, etc.

Over the last few decades, a steadily increasing number of children have been diagnosed with what used to be called "adult-onset diabetes." Kids are developing type 2 diabetes because they are eating foods loaded with far too much refined carbohydrate and becoming overweight at very young ages. The Smart for Life ThinAdventure program for kids is based on low glycemic foods. You can read more in the Bonus Section: ThinAdventure Healthy Weight Program for Kids.

4. You can choose to include our specially designed food products to help keep your hunger at bay and improve your overall health.

When patients come to Smart for Life Weight Management Centers, they usually choose to purchase some of our meal replacement products. Following the program is easier if you don't have to prepare all your own foods. So we make this simple for you by offering Smart for Life cookies, muffins, soups, protein bars, shakes, and beverages. All our products are 60% organic with no preservatives. We use triple-filtered water and add special health ingredients like omega-3 fatty acids, flaxseed, and powerful fibers.

Most of my patients fall in love with the Smart for Life cookies. These cookies are not like the cookies you buy at the supermarket. I developed these cookies in a food research laboratory, and it took me years of experimentation to discover the right ingredients that would taste great and allow for healthy weight loss.

Smart for Life cookies are specially formulated to be low glycemic foods. All our cookies are high in fiber and protein, two nutritional components that add value while working to reduce hunger. They are specially formulated to suppress hunger; in-fact they are patent-pending because of this process. Many of my patients tell me they work as well as prescription medication. We have a wide variety of flavors, including chocolate chip, oatmeal raisin, cranberry, blueberry, and banana chocolate chip granola. Some of our cookies are gluten-free for those with wheat allergies.

You can buy Smart for Life cookies by the box, or you can purchase the cookie mix and make the cookies yourself. On my website, you can find recipes for some of my Smart for Life cookies. That way, you can make the cookies yourself and save money. Unfortunately, you cannot add all of the special ingredients we are able to use in our products because some are not available commercially, such as our special fibers. So your homemade cookies may not pack the anti-hunger punch that ours do, but they should taste delicious, fill you up, and help you lose weight.

There are plenty of recipes on my website for Smart muffins, shakes, soups, and beverages as well. Again, you may choose to purchase our products or make your own. But do remember that we add some ingredients you won't find in the store, and these food components can provide an extra edge for dieters.

5. You will not start on an exercise program until you have your metabolism under control.

The advice not to rush to exercise usually comes as a surprise to my patients. But I know from personal experience as well as years of working with thousands of overweight people: *exercise makes us eat more.*

Physical activity stimulates the appetite. This is a normal

metabolic response to caloric expenditure. Appetite is part of a natural system to ensure the body replenishes caloric losses. But when we are trying to shed pounds, an increase in appetite becomes a problem. If you eat too much after exercising, which is a natural consequence to working out, exercise can prove self-defeating.

You'll read more on exercise in Chapter 4: The Smart for Life Exercise Program. In the meantime, please take my advice and refrain from starting on an exercise regimen until you have lost a good amount of the weight you need to lose. If you are already following a regular exercise routine, you can certainly continue on your program. Just don't increase your level of activity. Not yet. If you do, you'll find your appetite stimulated in response, and you'll want to eat more.

6. You will make a commitment to the program, and we will provide you with support and assistance throughout your diet journey.

I can share with you everything you need to know to lose all the weight you want to lose. But only you—*and you alone*—can make weight loss happen. You'll need to make a commitment to lose that weight. All you need to do is start. So, go ahead: just do it. Get started *right now.*

Some of my patients find it helps to write out a contract with themselves, stating that they are going to start the RCD today and stick with it until they reach their goal weight. You can make a contract, too. Simply add a few sentences at the bottom of your weekly weigh-in chart. Make a binding contract with yourself to stay on the program.

Staying committed early may be the most difficult step you take on your weight loss journey. Sometimes the first step is the hardest. So, if you need some moral support, come see us at a Smart for Life Weight Management Center or contact us via our website. Our contact information is included in the Appendix.

Eat When You are Hungry, Drink Lots of Water

While you are on the Smart for Life diet plan, it is important *only to eat when you feel physically hungry*. You might not want to eat breakfast until after you arrive at your office. Or you may find yourself eating snacks every few hours then avoiding food after dinner. You might eat a light snack at night; you might not. Your days will vary, and every individual is different. What is most important is this: You'll need to learn how to listen to your own body's hunger signals. Smart For Life program products are designed to replace your breakfast, lunch, and snacks while you are on your weight loss journey.

It is imperative you stop using the clock as a guide for when to eat. Losing the "three squares a day" mentality is an essential aspect of becoming Smart for Life. You can start right now by vowing to yourself *never to eat unless you are physically hungry*. Then stick to your vow. You'll be amazed at how accurate your body can be in signaling you when there is a need—a real *need*, not just a desire—for food.

If you are unable to read your body's hunger signals, eat your meals and snacks every two to three hours. After you follow this strict schedule for a few weeks, you will find that your body is telling you when you are hungry. You will have retrained your body's hunger mechanisms by eating small meals and snacks spaced evenly throughout the day. If you find you feel hungry all the time, you may need medication. Information on hunger control is provided in Chapter 2.

How to tell when you are needing food rather than craving food is something you must learn to eat in response to physical hunger rather than emotional urges. Everyone has different internal hunger messages, and you should become aware of yours. Some people hear their stomach growl; others have mild headaches or a kind of inner emptiness. Figure out what your hunger signal is and pay attention to it. Don't wait until you are ravenous before you eat. Feeding extreme hunger can be a recipe for disaster as hungry people will eat anything and everything, typically in excessive amounts.

Whenever you are eating a meal or snack, you'll need to learn how to *stop eating before you are full.* Learning to stop is another essential aspect of becoming Smart for Life. You'll need to learn how to identify the comfort zone between feeling hungry and feeling full. I like to compare the feeling to the gauge on the fuel tank in your car: You eat until your inner gauge reads somewhere between 1/4 full and 3/4 full.

Stopping eating when you are not quite full can be tricky at first. Ceasing eating before we are stuffed is not what we learn growing up. At least, I didn't. I was a member of the empty plate club. Empty plate—or no dessert. This training instilled in me the habit of eating everything I am served. It took a lot of conscious effort to change this old habit.

Start practicing: every time you sit down to eat, make a conscious effort to tune in to your body's signals. Are you hungry? What does that feel like? Now, eat slowly. Pay attention to your body. Eat a small amount and focus on each bite. Try to gauge when you are 1/4 full, 1/2 full, 3/4 full. Then stop. Never eat until you feel stuffed. Over-eating no longer works for you.

But do drink a lot of water. I tell my patients they should consume at least 64 ounces of water every day. This means drinking eight 8-ounce glasses of water. My patients usually like to remind themselves by filling two 32-ounce bottles or one 64-ounce jug each morning and making sure to drink the full amount over the course of the day.

Did you know that water is an essential nutrient? We need plenty of fresh water to help many important body functions work smoothly. Water also helps flush out the toxins you will be excreting as you drop pounds and improve the content of your daily food intake.

You may substitute tea or coffee, but filtered water is the best choice.

Don't buy small bottles of water if you can avoid doing so. All that plastic is wasteful and contributes to our environmental woes. I advise my patients to buy a simple water filter they can use at home so that they can purify their own water supply—for themselves and their families.

Some parts of the country have a good water supply. I don't live in one of those places, so I use a water filtration system in my own home. And we triple filter any water included in Smart for Life products to ensure absolute purity.

Destock Your Pantry

When I'm hungry, food calls to me. The kind of food I don't want to eat—fast foods, rich foods, junk foods and desserts—intrudes on my thoughts. I find myself daydreaming about my favorite foods like Oreos and chocolate cake. Such desires are distracting. When I'm trying to lose weight, hearing the siren call of doughnuts I know are in the cupboard is dangerous.

If these types of foods are in my pantry, and I let myself go hungry all day, guess what happens when I get home? Right: I will eat whatever foods have been calling to me. But if I don't have these kinds of foods on hand at home, I'll settle for something healthy.

My wife used to keep chocolate-covered almonds around the house in pretty glass bowls. They looked nice but proved to be one of my downfalls. I would arrive home hungry and tired, and those little candies would call to me. Do you know how much sugar, fat, and calories a handful—or two—of chocolate-covered almonds contain? (A small handful can contain as many as 230 calories with 15 grams of fat and a whopping 17 grams of sugar!). I was sabotaging my weight loss efforts all the time, almost unconsciously.

I tell my patients at the Smart for Life Weight Management Centers the first thing to do after you sign up for the program *is destock your pantry.*

The key to success on the Smart for Life diet plan is to put out of your mind all the food that normally calls to you. If you have a weakness for chocolate like I do, and you're aware that there is some chocolate candy in your pantry, then that food will call your name all day and all night long until you heed the call and eat it. Then, of course, you will feel bad. I know; I used to raid the pantry to quiet the voices. Until I destocked my own pantry.

Do not read this section and then ignore this part of the program. I urge—beg, *demand*—you go into your kitchen today and remove all those foods that call to you. Not the carrots and green veggies, the lean meats and canned tuna. No, you know what foods you need to get rid of; you know exactly which foods put the weight on.

Typically, eliminating danger foods will mean getting rid of all the foods you have a weakness for and tend to overeat like candy, sweets, desserts of all kinds, chips and other packaged snack foods, comfort foods and cold cuts, soft drinks and sweetened juices, beer and alcoholic beverages. All the items you crave, snack on, and stuff. You know the foods I mean.

Be strong by kicking the enticing, bad foods to the curb. It is important to your diet success, your physical health, your life. It is time to march into the kitchen, the pantry, the wet bar and pack up all those foods and beverages that will lure you back into your old ways of eating. Clear your pantry now!

After you pack up a box—or two or three—of the problem foods and drinks, you can do your second good deed for the day: why not donate the boxes to a local food bank or shelter? Give your entire pantry to your favorite charity organization. Those people can use the foods you don't need anymore.

If your family lives on convenience foods, sweets and snacks (all the foods that are not on your new diet plan), now is the time to recruit their help. Sit everybody down tonight and tell them you need to keep the house clean of that kind of food for a while. Your family should be happy to support you on your journey. They should want to help you reach your weight loss goal. And don't feel too guilty about your request. Eating healthy will be good for the spouse and kids, too.

If you find destocking does not work because there are foods that call to you that belong to somebody else in your house, I have a trick you can do. Buy yourself some small blank stickers and print on them: *Not for*_______. Print your own name on the dotted line. Whenever you see a bag of chips or a candy bar belonging to a roommate or family member, put one of your stickers on it. My little trick is second best to removing all temptation from your home.

Avoid Gastroporn

Have you noticed how many cooking shows there are on television these days? Be Smart, don't watch these shows. They tend to be food industry sponsored and will make you crave foods you are no longer eating.

Try to avoid being lured in by manufactured food trends, new restaurants, and top chefs. Avoid all the culinary magazines with the mouthwatering photos of rich dishes. Remember, out of sight will mean out of mind and an end to the temptation posed by unhealthy foods.

The current media obsession with food and cooking has been referred to as "gastroporn." I love the term because it encapsulates the wrong way our society is looking at food. With gastroporn, the focus is on the unattainable, the tempting, the sinful dishes we are not supposed to want but do rather than on food as an essential factor in obtaining the energy and the nutrition we need for good health.

The food industry is manipulating us, warping and then overselling food—one of life's basic necessities. This is gastroporn. And, in my view, their glorification of an unhealthy relationship to food is similar to what the pornography industry has done with sex.

Be Smart and stay away while you eat healthy and get lean.

You are Getting Smarter Already

So now you've done it: you have begun the Smart for Life diet plan. You've received your doctor's okay to start a healthy weight loss regimen. You've dared to step on the scale (give yourself a pat on the back for this), and you've selected a goal weight. You've recorded the information on a weight chart you are keeping on paper or on your computer. You've reviewed the main components of the diet, and you've destocked your pantry of temptation foods. You know you will need to learn how to eat when you're hungry and stop before you're full. You're committed to becoming in tune with your body's signals and to adhering to the other important guidelines for Smart eating. In fact, you've signed a contract with yourself stating that you will follow the program. And you've got 64 ounces of water set aside to drink during the next 24 hours.

Okay, great job.

But wait, you say. *What the heck am I supposed to eat on this diet?*

Good question. You can use the chart below to guide you as you begin your journey. As you read more chapters, you will become adept at selecting the foods that will help you to become metabolically efficient. For now, use the following guidelines:

In Chapter 6 you can get more details, but the chart below explains the program in a nut shell. You can make your own cookies at home, or buy them online or at a retailer near you. Because the cookies are made with unique ingredients which are not available at your local grocery store, we made these ingredients available on our website.

Day 1 – 7:

Every day you will choose from the following items for breakfast, lunch, and all snacks. Only your dinners will vary.

BREAKFAST
Smart for Life cookie, muffin, shake, cereal or other hunger-suppressing product

Midmorning SNACK
Smart for Life cookie, muffin, shake, cereal, soup or other hunger-suppressing product

LUNCH
Smart for Life cookie, muffin, shake, cereal, soup or other hunger-suppressing product

Midafternoon SNACK
Smart for Life cookie, muffin, shake, cereal, soup or other hunger-suppressing product

Late Afternoon SNACK
Smart for Life cookie, muffin, shake, cereal, soup or other hunger-suppressing product

Anytime Snack
Smart for Life cookie, muffin, shake, cereal, soup or other hunger-suppressing product

Day 1 – 7 Dinner:

Day 1 Dinner: Fish with Peppers, Tomatoes and Capers* and salad

Day 2 Dinner: Moroccan Turkey* and salad

Day 3 Dinner: Sautéed Chicken Breast with Artichokes and Peppers* and salad

Day 4 Dinner: Scallops with Capers and Tomatoes* and salad

Day 5 Dinner: Chopped Greek Salad with Chicken* and salad

Day 6 Dinner: Tilapia and Summer Vegetable Packets* and salad

Day 7 Dinner: Crab Cakes* and salad

All dinner meal must be accompanied with a vegetables or salad.
All dinners above with asterisk can be found in the recipe section of the book.

You can order the ingredients at www.smartforlife.com/drsassbook and all baking instructions will come with them. If you choose to do the program without cookies, please see the plan in chapter 6, but I assure you the cookies are the easiest and least expensive. You can bake two weeks worth in less then an hour and at a fraction of the cost of the food program. If you want to add functional ingredients to the cookies you can order those at: www.smartforlife.com/drsassbook as well.

Vegetables are Superfoods

We all know that vegetables are good for us. Veggies are rich sources of fiber, vitamins, and other nutrients. But most people don't realize that eating plenty of vegetables can help the body to turn on longevity genes.

Vegetables are naturally rich in microtoxins. These chemical substances help veggies to resist invasion by insects and fungi. Whenever we eat vegetable microtoxins, these invisible chemicals signal our bodies to turn on protective genes. This makes us resistant to harmful toxins, and provides us with increased resistance to cellular damage. The process is similar to vaccination, allowing the body to create a natural immunity to invaders that cause disease.

Vegetables can boost the immune system. Veggies help our cells to resist oxidation, which prevents premature aging. I call them Superfoods. Including Superfoods like vegetables in your daily diet can help you to live a long, healthy life.

At this point, I hand my patients our Smart for Life guidebook that outlines the spectrum of Smart Foods (and Wrong Foods). This is the next step in their weight loss journey. For those of you who are reading *Smart for Life*, however, I'm adding a brief side trip to the journey. I want to educate you about appetite and the drugs used to suppress it.

Then you can read Chapter 3: Smart Foods, and you will find out exactly what to eat so you may begin to lose weight, get healthy, and retrain your metabolism.

You are on your way to being Smart for Life.

Chapter 2: Smart (and not so smart) Weight Loss Tools

After the young Italian guy died on my watch in the ER, I had a kind of awakening. My eyes were suddenly opened to something I'd been blind to for years. I began to look around me at the hospital. A lot of the medical staff were overweight. The nurses were fat and so were the physicians in various departments.

We were all eating on the run, busy people grabbing fast foods and chowing down in the staff room, basically living on restaurant delivery. We weren't eating when we were hungry. We were stuffing tacos and pizza in whenever we had a chance, eating like we might never get the time for a meal again. That's how it feels when you're on the go, not eating regularly, and wildly stressed.

I began to notice how many of my patients were overweight. A lot of the people I treated were obese, and they invariably had all sorts of health problems directly related to their weight: insulin resistance, diabetes, high blood pressure, elevated blood lipids, metabolic syndrome, asthma, sleep apnea, gallbladder disorders, intestinal issues, depression.

What I realized was this: I had been thinking of my patients' diseases as the problem to be solved, but *it was obesity itself that was the problem. The common chronic disorders like diabetes and heart disease, these were the symptoms of obesity.*

The revelation occurred: I began to see the truth. We were a fat society. Because we were so fat, we were also an unhealthy culture.

I became acutely aware of the obesity epidemic impacting modern society. I saw the results every day in the emergency room and on the floors of the hospital. I noticed overweight people everywhere I went and in the media, older adults and teens, parents and young kids, everybody fat and unhealthy looking. As a society, we were growing fatter and fatter, and our health was suffering. Some of us were dying young because we were too fat.

My experiences in the emergency room influenced me in a way

that would decide the course of my career. First, I became determined to lose weight myself and keep the pounds off.

Losing the weight I had gained proved more difficult than I had ever imagined.

I needed to lose around 40 pounds. Forty pounds didn't seem like a big challenge at first. I thought I would simply exercise more, and the weight would just disappear.

I signed up at a local gym and began going every other day for an hour or an hour and a half. Pretty soon I felt tighter, more healthy, and more fit. But it was next to impossible for me to maintain the exercise regimen. I was a busy doctor, and life got in the way. Plus, after six months of working out all the time and sweating and making the effort, I hadn't lost any weight. Not a single pound.

At the time, I was not aware of the massive amount of literature showing that exercise alone is not an efficient way to lose weight. The math on this is simple. If you need to burn 3500 calories to lose a pound of body fat, and one or two hours of exercise only burns maybe 500 calories, one would need to spend a couple of hours a day in the gym for a whole week to lose a single pound. It is very difficult to pull off such extreme exercise routines week after week, no matter how determined we might be to get in shape.

And there's the annoying fact that exercise increases the appetite. People who work out tend to replace the burned calories with increased food intake. I know I did. All I had to do to counteract any weight loss from exercise was to eat a couple of slices of pizza or some eggrolls in the staff room, and that was all too easy for me to do.

In fact, I found I was exercising and then eating more and then exercising to burn up the extra calories I had taken in. It was a silly cycle, a vicious circle. And I wasn't losing weight. Even though I was trying to follow the medical mantra of the time, which was "eat less, exercise more," I could only exercise more. I found I couldn't eat less because I was hungry.

Even though I was getting in shape, I didn't look trim. My belly was too round. I looked at myself in the mirrors at the gym, and there was no denying I was fat. If you had seen me walking by on the street, you would have considered me fat. My BMI was 31 or 32, which as you know from Chapter 1 is in the range that the medical profession regards as obese.

I was fat all right. My BMI was greater than my age. But I regarded my extra pounds as a temporary condition. I was very determined to lose weight. I knew I would succeed. It was simply a question of how. I remember thinking at the time: *how can I eat so that I will lose weight and not be hungry all the time, so hungry that I eat the foods I know are piling on the pounds?*

Appetite and Hunger

The most important weight loss tools you have are your attitude and your commitment. If you have a positive attitude and believe you can lose weight, you will lose weight. If you make a commitment to the Smart for Life program and stick with it, then you will succeed. You will successfully lose weight.

However, some additional tools may be necessary. I certainly needed more than my positive attitude toward losing weight and my strong commitment to change. What I needed was something to help me feel less hungry so that I could *control my appetite.*

It took me a long time to find the help I needed. Over the years, I have discovered helpful (and not so helpful) weight loss medications and products. After years of research and work with thousands of patients, I discovered what I will share with you here. I am constantly looking for more tools, new and improved products that I can utilize—safely and successfully—for myself and with my patients.

Let me share with you what I currently tell my patients about at the Smart for Life Weight Management Centers. The medications and special food ingredients I like to use with my patients may help you to get a kick-start on your weight loss endeavors. Or, if you reach a weight plateau and find you just can't shed the pounds you need to drop, the following information may prove helpful.

When my patients embark on the Smart for Life program, most of them begin right away to lose weight. But a minority discover they are just too hungry on the diet. Their appetite is overriding their desire to eat healthfully. They actually feel hunger, physical hunger (not emotional craving), between meals or even immediately after eating.

If a patient tells me he or she cannot follow the program because of hunger, I offer them tools to help retrain the appetite. Note that some of these products are available on our website while others require a prescription. The prescription drugs mandate medical monitoring to prevent illness, allergic reactions, or serious side effects. Dieters who visit a Smart for Life Weight Management Center can ask about prescriptions for appetite suppressants because all of our patients are medically supervised. Of course, you can see your own family doctor or bariatric physician.

Your doctor may be helping you to manage the results of your excess weight, the diseases and dysfunctions. But now you are willing to confront the *causes* of your excess weight. You are willing to get to the root of the problem. Tell your doctor how he or she can help you. If necessary, inform your doctor that you will need a prescription appetite suppressant.

Appetite Suppressants

During the 1990s, a popular appetite suppressant called Fen-phen was removed from the market because of serious, potentially life-threatening side effects. Since that time, appetite suppressants in general have been regarded skeptically. Even if made from entirely safe ingredients, appetite suppressants continue to have a bad rap.

But let's be clear: some overweight people need appetite suppressants just as some people cannot control their blood pressure unless they use blood pressure medication, and others need medication to control blood cholesterol or insulin levels. The same physiological need exists in certain cases of obesity: without appetite suppressant medication, hunger and appetite regulatory mechanisms are out of control.

I find that perhaps one out of every five patients I see at the Smart for Life Weight Management Centers needs an appetite suppressant medication to start their weight loss process. I look at these medications as Smart tools on the road to weight loss success. Our cookies and other products contain natural appetite suppressing ingredients, so these natural ingredients works for the majority of people. But for some, extra help is required. They are hungry on the RCD, go off the diet plan, and fail to lose weight. When weight loss is not happening, I prescribe one or another of the few medications I know to be both safe and effective.

Here's how to tell if you need appetite suppressants: begin on the RCD provided in the next chapter. Try the program for two weeks. Did you fail to lose any weight? Were you hungry all the time? Did you find yourself eating foods not included on the diet because you were ravenous? If your answers to these questions are *yes*, you might want to try an appetite suppressant.

When one of my patients is having hunger issues while on the Smart for Life program, I will suggest HungerBlock. This natural product is available at the Smart for Life Weight Management Centers and on our website. Made with egg-white protein and other natural ingredients, HungerBlock will help curb your appetite so you can remain on the diet long enough to correct your body's imbalanced appetite control mechanism.

So, if you aren't having success on the RCD plan, try HungerBlock for a week and see if that does the trick. Give this specially designed weight loss tool at least a week to see if your appetite begins to realign itself with your body's actual need for food.

If HungerBlock doesn't help you stick to the program, you may need a prescription appetite suppressant, which means you'll need to be under medical supervision.

First, you will need to get certain medical tests. You can schedule a visit with your own physician or go to a Smart for Life Weight Management Center. You can make an appointment with a bariatric physician who is a member of the American Society of Bariatric Physicians. You can check online to find a qualified bariatrician in your area. If you are in South Florida, you can come see me.

You will need to get an EKG test and a physical exam to make sure there are no heart irregularities that would preclude the use of appetite suppressants. You'll also need a blood test. If medically approved, you will receive the green light to use appetite suppressant drugs.

Remember, you MUST use the medication in conjunction with a sound weight loss program. If you take an appetite suppressant and continue to eat the way you have been, then the drug will do nothing. Not changing your habits is a waste of time and money. You must use the drug while adhering to a weight loss diet plan like the one in *Smart for Life.*

Prescription Suppressants

The only two prescription appetite suppressants I prescribe for my patients are Phendertamerazine and Phentramine. These two medications are safe when used judiciously under medical supervision.

Although you can buy them illegally on the Internet, I advise my patients not to do so. *You need to have a qualified physician monitoring you during the use of these two drugs, either your own doctor or one at a Smart for Life center. This is the only safe way to take these two medications.*

These drugs only work if your body needs them. You must find out whether you actually need them before you take them. Be sure to make an appointment with a qualified physician and find out if you are a candidate before you get a prescription for these medications.

Metformin

Another weight loss medication I use with some of my patients is Metformin, a drug that works to correct insulin resistance. Many overweight people are suffering from insulin resistance, which contributes to an inability to reduce food intake and causes a continuous increase in the storage of body fat. There is more information on insulin resistance in Chapter 8 for those readers who wish to learn about this increasingly common metabolic imbalance.

Insulin resistance is the first stage of diabetes. Once your cells become resistant to insulin, you are on your way to becoming diabetic.

If you are insulin resistant, your blood sugar remains elevated because most of your body's cells cannot use the circulating blood sugar (glucose). Your fat cells, however, do not become insulin resistant, so these cells continue to store the circulating glucose and convert it to body fat. The rest of your body's cells are not receiving the energy they need for proper function. You feel tired and unwell. You're hungry. Your body produces more insulin, but the increased production does no good. You become increasingly insulin resistant. You feel worse every day. You get fatter and fatter.

This is the vicious cycle of insulin resistance. Unchecked, the process will continue until you develop diabetes.

A sound weight loss program that results in significant weight loss will reduce and eventually reverse insulin resistance. However, some of my patients need a prescription to jump-start the process. Being insulin resistant makes you hungry and tired. Sometimes you need more than what the diet can provide so your body is not too hungry and you do not become easily discouraged.

The only medication I know that decreases insulin resistance significantly and does not cause weight gain is Metformin. If you take insulin instead, your insulin resistance will get worse. DO NOT TAKE INSULIN for insulin resistance. Insulin as a prescription should be used only if your body no longer makes insulin. If you are insulin resistant, your body may have a perfectly adequate insulin supply. But with insulin resistance, your cells are no longer able to utilize the insulin supply properly. Taking insulin will not help the imbalance. In fact, taking insulin will make you fatter.

However, if you are taking insulin because your doctor has prescribed it, do not stop unless your doctor approves a new treatment plan for you. *Always consult your physician before making any changes in the use of prescription medications.*

Metformin can help with insulin resistance. There are some studies indicating that Metformin also has anti-aging properties. Research is being conducted to investigate how Metformin might slow the aging process and how insulin resistance may make you age faster. The connection makes sense. We already know an imbalance in your body's glucose storage mechanisms leads to disease. Aging accelerates when your body is unhealthy.

When my patients take Metformin, they begin to feel better even before the weight comes off. They have more energy, their hunger diminishes, and they are able to follow the RCD plan. They find that sometimes for the first time ever, they are able to lose weight, and they are able to maintain their weight loss.

Metformin should only be used under medical supervision. You can ask your own physician about Metformin. He or she should be able to give you a simple blood test and, if needed, a prescription for this safe and effective drug. Because more than 20% of Americans are insulin resistant, and around 50% of obese individuals may be insulin resistant, you should have the test to see if insulin resistance is a problem for you.

I feel strongly about this: if you need a prescription drug to help you lose weight, your doctor should be willing to prescribe one for you. Obesity is a significant threat to your life. *Being fat is dangerous.*

Today's doctors need to become acutely aware of this fact and keep abreast of the scientific research so they can assist their overweight patients safely, successfully to lose excess weight.

Here is a story that will blow your mind. Katrina H. was headed for an early demise before she lost weight with Smart for Life.

Katrina H.

When she walked, her whole body hurt. She was so overweight, she could not get up from a chair or arise from her bed without suffering pain in her bones, muscles, and joints. Her breathing was labored, her legs were swollen—and she wasn't even a senior citizen yet.

Katrina H. was worried about her future. Even her doctor was worried. He warned her that if she didn't lose around 100 pounds, she would soon find herself confined to a wheelchair.

That scared Katrina. But she wasn't sure how to shed all the pounds her doctor told her she had to lose. And her doctor did not tell her *how* to lose the life-threatening weight.

Fortunately, she remembered seeing a sign or an advertisement for a weight loss program near where she lived in Canada. One day Katrina drove to the Smart for Life Weight Management Center and signed up.

In less than a year, Katrina lost 95 pounds.

"I wrote everything down," Katrina remembers. She discussed her issues with the staff at the Center, and they gave her the feedback she needed to remain on the program. Katrina learned how to eat a more balanced diet. "You have to follow the program," she advises others who want to lose weight. "But if I can follow it, anyone can. I have had weight issues all my life. This was the first time in all my life that I ever reached my goals."

After the pounds came off, she began to feel better than she had in years. Her knees didn't hurt. She could get up and around more easily. She could breathe again. On a whim, Katrina signed up for an aerobics class. Then she discovered that she really liked taking brisk walks. She felt good about eating healthy foods every day and feeding her family better.

These days, Katrina H. feels good about her future. "The key for me is to live a good life, and a healthier life, so I can be around for my grandkids," she says.

And that's exactly what she is doing.

Some Not so Helpful Tools

Whatever you do, avoid all the diet fads. I tried many of them, and you will read about what a waste of time that was for me. See, I know how you feel: you desperately want to lose weight, so you are willing to eat only grapefruit and cottage cheese or just drink some chemical-laden "diet" liquid that comes in cans. You'll do just about anything to lose the weight. I was like this once myself.

But come on. You know the facts as well as I do: these fad diets never work. You may lose a few pounds only to regain the weight as soon as you begin eating normally again. And that's just it: you *will* eat normally again—or whatever constitutes "normal" for you—which means you'll return to eating a lot of the foods that add pounds and not enough of the foods that help to create an efficient metabolism.

So please, do yourself a favor: avoid all diet fads. These fads will not suppress your appetite. They will increase your hunger for inappropriate foods because while your body is lacking in the calories and nutrients it needs for proper function, your cells will be getting the wrong messages. And you know what that means: your body will remain inefficient. You'll store lots of fat. And you'll feel hungry.

Personally, I'm not a fan of over-the-counter weight loss aids like Alli. These products tend to be little more than fads. Like fad diets, they do nothing to help you change your eating habits and your metabolism. Save your money. Spend it on healthy food.

If you haven't figured this out already, I'm a fan of natural food. The closer a food is to the way Mother Nature prepares it, the more I like it. I believe our bodies readily digest and absorb the essential nutrients available in natural foods while our cells and organs are not sure what to do with the chemicals, preservatives, food dyes, and other artificial ingredients in a lot of modern foods. Most of the diet products sold today are loaded with these unnatural ingredients. Over-processed foods are not good for you, and fad diets based on them will not help you permanently to lose the weight you want to lose.

Medications that Add Weight

Before you begin on the Smart for Life program, you might want to take a look at the following list of prescription medications that interfere with weight loss. Some of these drugs cause water retention, and others stimulate the appetite. Some actually create metabolic changes that lead to increased fat storage and weight gain.

If you are taking any of these medications, be aware of the influence on your weight. You can discuss the implications with your doctor.

Note that after significant weight is lost, medication dosages may need to be adjusted for any drugs you might be taking. Some of my patients are able to discontinue their prescription drug use once a healthy weight is attained.

Drugs that Cause Weight Gain

Diabetes drugs:

Insulin

Thiazolidinediones

Sulfonylureas

Steroid hormones:

Corticosteroids

Progestational steroids

Psychiatric/neurologic drugs:

Antidepressants (Tricyclic Antidepressants, Selective Serotonin Reuptake Inhibitors, Monoamine Oxidase Inhibitors, Lithium)

Antipsychotics

Anticonvulsants

Miscellaneous drugs:

Antihistamines

Alpha-adrenergic blockers

Beta-adrenergic blockers

Smart Foodstuffs

In case you decide to try some of the Smart for Life products, I want you to know about our special ingredients. These ingredients are called "functional foods" because they have special health-related functions in the body.

All of our functional ingredients have been carefully designed to enhance your success on the Smart for Life program. These ingredients are good for your body because they regulate your blood sugar, blood lipids, and cholesterol and aid digestive health and/or help send messages to your body's cells to improve your metabolic efficiency. All of these ingredients have been tested on humans in scientifically designed studies to determine safety and efficacy. All of these functional products are safe, and they really work.

1. LeptiCore
2. ThinAdventure Fiber
3. plant sterols
4. inulin
5. natural sweeteners
6. fish oil
7. flaxseed

LeptiCore is a functional ingredient used in some of our cookies. You won't taste it, but you will notice a difference. LeptiCore has been specially formulated to reduce your body's leptin resistance.

A recently discovered hormone, leptin regulates body fat storage by influencing appetite and metabolism. Overweight people tend to have high levels of leptin in the blood, but they are resistant to its effects. This is similar to insulin resistance. With leptin resistance, LeptiCore fixes the problem. By enhancing the function of leptin in your body, LeptiCore helps reduce your appetite, boost your metabolism, and minimize fat storage. More on the science behind this interesting hormone in Chapter 8.

ThinAdventure Fiber is an incredibly effective source of dietary fiber. Intake of this high-powered mega-fiber helps to regulate blood sugar, insulin, and appetite. This special fiber is also influential in reducing elevated blood lipids including cholesterol.

Numerous medical studies have shown that high fiber diets help to lower blood lipids significantly, and fiber is important in digestive health. ThinAdventure Fiber is a super-fiber that is super efficient in achieving these healthy effects. This is why we use ThinAdventure Fiber in some of our products.

Plant sterols, also known as phytosterols, occur naturally in plants. They can be used in supplement form to lower blood cholesterol. According to the Food and Drug Administration, plant sterols can lower the risk of heart disease. This is why we add plant sterols to our products.

Inulin is a kind of fiber found naturally in root vegetables. Onions, garlic, wild yam, chicory, agave, and certain other roots are rich in inulin. It is mildly sweet and has a low glycemic index. Some studies indicate that inulin may lower blood lipids. However, we add it to our products because it adds a sweet flavor, is an excellent fiber, and is good for the intestines.

Natural sweeteners like inulin are preferable to sugar. There are many reasons for this including the fact that sugar is about as high on the glycemic index as a foodstuff can get. High sugar intakes cause wild swings in blood glucose and insulin. Sugar—and its relatives corn sweeteners and fructose—are massively overused by the food industry to make foods taste good so we'll overeat them. Sugar is, in my opinion, one of the main causes of our obesity and diabetes epidemics. At Smart for Life, we prefer natural sweeteners like stevia.

But, you say, *sugar is sort of natural.* After all, it comes from sugarcane, which is a plant. Right? Yes, but. But what they do to the sugarcane to turn it into the world's most popular sweetener is incredible. To summarize, the manufacturers remove all the nutrient-rich parts of the plant and process the heck out of it until all that is left are those sweet, white granules.

And the effect on the body is remarkable: Sugar elevates the body's blood glucose very rapidly, triggering an insulin response. If, like most overweight people, your body has become insulin resistant, sugar is sending the wrong messages to your body's cells. All that processed sugar is making your body metabolically inefficient and fat. Even moderately high sugar intakes set you on the road to type 2 diabetes and other chronic diseases.

Recent research has indicated that fructose can be even more unhealthy. Cheaper than white sugar, fructose-based sweeteners made from corn were introduced into many processed foods during the 1980s. High-fructose corn syrup (HFCS) replaced regular sugar in many foods and beverages, including soft drinks. However, fructose is metabolized differently than regular sugar and may have an undesirable impact on the liver. Medical researchers believe high intakes of fructose can cause fat to build up in the liver, leading to illness and disease. Fructose also can cause insulin resistance. Plus, the way fructose is metabolized in the body increases your appetite.

In a word, DON'T EAT SUGAR or corn sweeteners like HFCS. If you need to sweeten your foods, try a little stevia, which comes from an herb. If you can't stand the taste of stevia, you might use Splenda. It's not very natural, but it will sweeten your food without caloric consequences and with minimal health effects.

Better yet, learn to appreciate the natural flavor of foods. Once you allow your taste buds to appreciate real food flavors, you may find that you do not need to add any sweeteners at all.

Fish oil is an excellent source of omega-3 fatty acids, essential fats abundant in cold water fish like sardines, bluefish, mackerel, and wild salmon. These fats help build hormones and other anti-inflammatory products in the body. Research has shown that diets low in omega-3 fatty acids can result in depression, heart disease, and a variety of inflammatory diseases like arthritis, asthma, and eczema. Regular intake of fish oils may reduce these and other conditions and can help to improve cardiovascular function.

All of us need to include adequate amounts of omega-3 fatty acids in our diets, but these fats are not found in the processed foods most people are consuming these days. That's why fish oils have been added to some Smart for Life products. Fish oils can be fishy smelling, but we use an odorless form as a truly healthy addition to some of our cookies. If you want to take a fish oil supplement, make sure to ingest at least 2000 mg daily.

Flaxseed is another functional food included in Smart for Life products. Like fish oil, flaxseed is a rich source of omega-3 fatty acids. You will read more about this amazing food in Chapter 3: Smart Foods because I regard flaxseed as a Superfood, one that can contribute to weight loss as well as overall health.

You can order these ingredients to add to your home baked cookies or other baked goods to add healthy, functional ingredients at www.smartforlife.com/drsassbook.

Supplements

When patients begin on the Smart for Life program, I advise them to take nutrition supplements. Supplements are nutritional insurance, a way to be sure essential nutrients are included in the diet every day. Usually I advise my patients to start taking a daily multivitamin and mineral supplement, one of the many affordable products they might buy in a health food store or local pharmacy. I tell them to take vitamin D-3 as well.

I also suggest taking probiotics. I'm a fan of intestinal health, and probiotics are key. The best probiotic supplements can be found in the refrigerated section of the local health food store.

Probiotics are live bacteria, including but not limited to the bacteria found in yogurt and other fermented products. This good bacteria is needed for healthy intestinal function. You'll read more about how important intestinal funtion is to weight loss as well as overall health in Chapter 8, but let me say this right now: take probiotics, and your body will begin to digest and eliminate properly.

Some of my patients take additional supplements like calcium and iron but only if they need to. You can always discuss nutrition supplementation with your physician. If you need more information on supplements, appetite suppressants, or functional foods, feel free to contact us by phone or through our website. See the Appendix for our contact information.

Here's another Smart for Life success story to inspire you before you read Chapter 3: Smart Foods. This story always brings a smile to my face.

Patsy C.

"I was always the fat, funny friend," Patsy C. says. You know the type. We've all had them or been them. By the time she was 25 years old, Patsy weighed 280 pounds. She was funny but only with her friends. "I was afraid to eat in public. I hated beach trips and was a lover of everything elastic. I was always single," Patsy recalls. "I had started to think that being overweight would always be my life."

Patsy wanted to enjoy her life without the constant mental and physical strain of being overweight. She felt like others were judging her, and that made her feel bad about herself. She knew that her excess weight made her unhealthy. Heart disease and diabetes were issues in her family, and this concerned Patsy. She worried constantly. Clothes that looked good on her were hard to find. "Being overweight is a full time job," Patsy C. says, "and I was done with it."

From the age of 10, Patsy had tried to lose weight. And she had tried everything, every fad diet she heard about. Patsy admits she once ate an all meat diet. She drank special diet shakes; she ate only vegetables. For a while, she ate all her meals before 5 p.m. "Nothing worked," she recalls. Then she heard about Smart for Life.

"I started on yet another diet journey," Patsy C. remembers. "But this diet was unlike the many I had tried before." The Smart for Life diet was healthy, filling, and nutritionally balanced. And satisfying. "Starving yourself, only drinking your meals, eating only raw vegetables... This is not smart. And that's why the other diets never worked for me," Patsy says now. "The good thing about Smart for

Life is it's just that: Smart for our lives."

Patsy learned how to eat differently from Smart for Life support staff. "They taught me the importance of eating smaller meals throughout the day, which was a vital part of my weight loss. In two weeks, I lost over 7 pounds, which was exactly the motivation I needed to continue on the program." She liked the food, and the Smart for Life products fit her lifestyle. "They are great for an on-the-go healthy snack that actually fills me up."

Patsy followed the program for 14 months straight. During this time, she lost 105 pounds.

"Overall, I'm a very healthy person. I work out every day now. My entire body has improved. I feel better on the outside and on the inside," Patsy says. "I'm in a completely different place than I was 3 years ago thanks to Smart for Life. My family and friends are all very impressed and proud. They were all a great help during my weight loss journey. Many of them are now Smart for Life fans as well."

Patsy wants to lose another 30 pounds. "Working out leads me to consume more calories, so I just need to make sure I'm eating the right things. Even if it's healthier foods, I need to watch what I eat," she says. Last time we talked, she was back on the RCD and expected to lose the additional pounds by the end of the summer.

Patsy C. is still the funny friend. But now she's the happy, confident, very attractive friend. "Now I am the funny friend who loves to go shopping and never turns down a beach trip," she says. "My life has done a 180! I'm so much happier, confident, and active. I don't have the urges I once did for food because I would never want to allow myself to be so overweight again. The changes in every aspect of my life are indescribable. I never knew how different my life would be once the weight came off."

Chapter 3: Smart Foods

When I was trying to lose weight as a young overweight doctor, I didn't try to change my diet. Not at first. I continued to eat in the staff room, all the wrong foods and too much of them while exercising as much as possible. I tried swimming, then karate. I kept going to the gym. I was on the treadmill whenever I had time to run.

I did not lose weight. I was hungry. I ate more and exercised more.

Finally, I quit exercising altogether. I decided I had to focus on my food intake instead.

I thought the best idea would be to cut down on food. Drastically. In fact, I was determined to fast once a week for an entire day. I expected the weight would slide right off if I was strong enough not to eat. Besides, I had begun to examine the medical literature about weight and health. I read some studies that suggested people who fast might live longer. How bad could not eating be?

Pretty bad, it turned out. I starved myself one day a week. Each time, I lost a couple of pounds. But as soon as I began eating again the next day, the weight would return. I ate more because I was hungry.

After a day without food, I would wake up ravenous. My body was in control and would not allow me to skimp on food intake. My favorite foods kept calling to me, calling my name. "Dr. Sass, come enjoy this piece of cake," I would hear. And my stomach felt so empty. What could I do? Oreos and chocolate-covered almonds were beckoning to me. And I was truly hungry!

Fasting lasted a month or so. I next tried a liquid diet. This only lasted a few days. The beverage tasted horrible. I could barely get it down. How could I function at work all day while only drinking that chalky, fake-tasting stuff? A liquid meal replacement diet was not for me.

Next I joined a weight loss group program, the kind where you come in to get weighed on a regular basis and share your difficulties with counselors or other dieters. Wow, was that diet complicated. There was a point system associated with the foods, and special preparation was required. It was a lot of work, and the weight loss was slow. After 5 or 6 weeks, I had only lost 5 pounds. I was not impressed. Too much effort for very little result.

A commercial meal replacement diet sounded like something that might fit my hectic lifestyle. I decided to try a program where I had no choice in foods. The only food I would eat was the commercial diet product the program sold.

I started on a plan with high hopes. My hopes and my commitment to the program lasted a very short while. Once I tasted the food and realized it didn't taste like food at all, I quit.

Most commercial diet foods and beverages are made with lots of additives, preservatives, salt, sugar, and artificial sweeteners. A lot of these products are shelf-stable, meaning that the foods can sit in your pantry for years and not become stale. Imagine the amount of preservatives it takes to keep chicken or fish from going bad without refrigeration. The companies that make these foods want to prepare as much product as possible as cheaply as possible and keep it on store shelves for as long as possible. That's how they make the biggest profit.

Personally, I like to know what's in the food I eat. I like to eat food that is as natural as possible. The diet food I was eating on the commercial meal replacement program seemed closer in construction (and taste) to cardboard than real food. It didn't even look like real food. I wasn't an astronaut; I didn't need food that could last for years in outer space.

By this time, I had become discouraged with my weight loss failures. I felt like I had tried everything, but nothing had worked for me. I was more fit, but I remained fat.

Something needed to be done, and I knew I would be the one that had to do it. But what?

On the Smart for Life program, you won't have to go through all the failure I experienced before you achieve permanent weight loss success. I've already done all the experimenting for you. If you've already tried all the exercise programs and weight loss diets out there, but you still are overweight and unhappy about it, I know how that feels, too.

So let me tell you something: the try and fail part of your life is over.

Smart for Life is where you begin to change the situation for good. This is where you begin to embark on your journey to become fit, trim, and Smart for Life.

By now, you have chosen your weight goal. You are committed to adopting the RCD, and your pantry has been destocked. Now all you need to know is what to eat and what not to eat: what's on the menu and what's off the menu.

To simplify this step on your journey, I've prepared some food lists for you. While you are on the RCD, select only those foods included on the Smart Foods list. Avoid all other foods. *If you don't see it here, don't eat it.* Not right now, not while you are trying to retrain your body to develop a more efficient metabolism.

I'm also including a list of Wrong Foods. These foods are NOT on your menu anymore—at least not now not while you are trying to lose weight. Later on, once you have reached your healthy weight goal, once your body is no longer storing too much food energy as fat, then you may learn how to include some of these Wrong Foods on an occasional basis. But for now, stay away. These foods will only spell trouble for you. They will serve as a giant obstacle on the road to weight loss success.

The third list I'm giving you here includes those foods I believe pack the most health for the least calories. I call these foods Superfoods. The Superfoods below are rich in nutrients like vitamins and minerals as well as other healthy factors like antioxidants, omega-3 fatty acids, and fiber. These foods send the right messages to your body's cells, boosting your overall health while helping you to lose excess body fat. Studies indicate that a diet rich in such Superfoods may improve resistance to disease and possibly increase longevity.

Notice that none of the Superfoods appear on the Wrong Foods list, but you probably guessed that.

Smart Foods

Vegetables

These foods may be served raw, steamed, boiled, roasted, sautéed, or baked.

artichokes

arugula

asparagus

bamboo

beets

bok choy

broccoli

Brussels sprouts

cabbage

carrots

cauliflower

celery

chard

chicory

chives

collards

cucumber

edamame

eggplant

endive

escarole

garlic

green beans

greens—including beet, collards, mustard, turnip

jicama

kale

leeks

lettuce

mushrooms

okra

onions

parsley

peas

peapods

peppers—green, red, yellow

pumpkin

purslane

radicchio

radishes

rhubarb

scallions

sea vegetables, seaweed

shallots

snow peas

spinach

sprouts

squash

Swiss chard

tomatoes, tomato puree

turnips

waterchestnuts

watercress

zucchini

Protein Foods

The following foods may be baked, steamed, broiled, poached, or grilled.

Fish—any fish including anchovies, bass, bluefish, carp, catfish, cod, flounder, grouper, haddock, halibut, herring, mackerel, mahi mahi, perch, pike, pollock, pompano, rockfish, salmon, sardines, skate, snapper, sole, sturgeon, swordfish, tilapia, trout, bluefish tuna, whitefish, whiting. Buy fresh or canned in water; no fried fish.

Shellfish—any shellfish including calamari, clams, conch, crab, crayfish, lobster, mussels, oysters, scallops, shrimp. Buy fresh or canned in water; no fried seafood

Poultry—chicken or turkey without skin, ground turkey, canned chicken in water, natural low-salt deli chicken and turkey without preservatives

Red meat—if you must include red meats, choose only wild meats like buffalo, venison, ostrich

Legumes—black, red, soy, pinto; chickpeas, lentils, split peas; hummus; tofu tempeh, miso

Egg whites (9-11 small egg whites are the equivalent of 6 ounces of lean protein)

Cheese—look for varieties that offer 0% total fat, less than 2 grams carbohydrate, and at least 5 grams of protein like Borden and Kraft low-fat cheeses, low-fat cottage cheeses, and low-fat soy cheeses

Milk—low-fat or skim milk, yogurt, soy milk, kefir; no chocolate or other flavored versions

Nuts—raw, unroasted, unsalted; almonds, cashews, walnuts are best; also almond milk; unroasted, unsalted pumpkin seeds and other seeds are fine too

Protein powders—soy, whey, hemp

High protein cereals—kashi, muesli, old-fashioned oats, ThinAdventure cereals, Kay's Naturals cereals

Other Foods

Dressings—olive oil, canola oil, vinegar

Condiments—capers, catsup, cocktail sauce, herbs, horseradish, hot sauce, fat-free mayonnaise, mustard, salsa, sea salt, soy sauce, spices, teriyaki sauce, Worcestershire sauce; use sparingly and look for unsweetened, low-sodium options

Club soda, tea, coffee

Also—flaxseeds; avocado; olives; sauerkraut, kimchi (fermented vegetables); fresh berries and other fruits in small quantities

Wrong Foods

Vegetables

No fried vegetables

No processed vegetable products made with added sauces or preservatives

No potatoes, sweet potatoes, fried potatoes, hash browns, etc.

Protein Foods

No beef, lamb, veal, or pork

No processed red meats or deli meats including salami, pepperoni, bologna, hot dogs, bacon, sausage

No fried meats or seafood; no frozen battered seafood or fish

No processed cheeses or cheese foods; no high-fat cheeses

No egg yolks

No flavored yogurts, no high-fat milk products, ice cream, frozen yogurt, cream, creamers

No roasted or salted nuts

Other Foods

No processed shelf-stable foods including convenience foods and microwavable items

No fast foods, over-processed snack foods

No soft drinks, sweetened drinks like lemonade, iced tea

No candy, cake, doughnuts, Danish, pastry, desserts

No cereals, breads, pastas, rice

No fruit juices

No sugar, honey, molasses, fructose, dextrose

No artificial creamers (Zilch creamer is ok because it has zero calories)

No chewing gum, breath mints, cough drops

No alcoholic beverages

Superfoods

Almonds: in the raw form, these delicious nuts are heart healthy with good fats, fiber, and the ability to lower blood cholesterol; almond milk is refreshing and naturally sweet

Pomegranates: rich in antioxidants, this fruit and the juice made from it has been shown to improve cardiac function in patients with heart disease

Kale: easily the most overlooked green vegetable, brimming with nutrients and fiber, antioxidants, and even protein; delicious in salads

Blueberries: rich in antioxidants, vitamins, and fiber, these delicious berries are not too sweet and easy to eat—alone or in shakes or recipes

Sprouts: rich in nutrients and fiber, add them to salads, an egg white omelet, or eat alone for a crunchy snack

Flaxseed: rich in omega-3 fatty acids; add to recipes, shakes, salads, or crackers

Fish: fresh fish is an excellent source of protein and omega-3 fatty acids; oily fish is higher in heart healthy fish oils than lean white fish; fatty fish lowest in mercury content include anchovies, herring, Atlantic mackerel, salmon, Atlantic sardines, sturgeon, and fresh bluefish tuna

Buffalo steak: no red meat is best, but if you must, this wild game meat is a better choice than most because the animals are more naturally raised, not fatted or corn-fed; eat sparingly, no more than once a week

Note: Superfoods are best when grown organically and/or produced locally.

I like these Superfoods as quick snacks: a handful of almonds or blueberries, a little bowl of sprouts or sliced pomegranate pieces. I try to include Superfoods regularly in my diet for their health-boosting antioxidants and other anti-aging factors.

Buy flaxseed and start adding it to your soups and salads, shakes, and other recipes. Include raw or cooked kale every week. Add it to your salads to boost the nutrient content. Put fresh fish on the menu regularly. If you are hooked on red meat, switch to buffalo steak. You won't believe how much better it tastes than industry produced beef.

Eating Naturally

You might have noticed something striking while looking at the lists above: all of the items on the Smart Foods and Superfoods lists are natural foods. That is, these foods are as close to the way Mother Nature made them as we can find. Each of these foods is unprocessed or minimally processed. This means these foods offer you healthy nutrition without any added artificial ingredients.

In general, if a food is in its natural state, there is only one ingredient: the food itself. A green bean. A slice of lean turkey. An egg white. A scallop. You see what I mean: natural, un-tampered with, whole foods. If we could live on foods like this, none of us would have a weight problem.

However, in today's modern world with our centralized food industry and 24/7 lifestyles, it is difficult to eat whole, natural foods all the time. For some of us, it's impossible. I understand the difficulty, believe me. So what I am asking you to do on the Smart for Life program is to be aware of the natural, whole foods available to you and eat them whenever you can. Choose less processed foods, more whole foods.

This is one of the reasons we make our own weight loss products. All of our foods and beverages at Smart for Life are minimally processed to retain the naturally high nutritional values while providing good taste and convenience. Smart for Life foods can be taken with you and eaten on the run. Smart for Life products are convenient foods that are not convenience foods because our foods are not over-processed.

In fact, when we manufacture our products, we use a special mixing technique that allows for very light processing. We blend the liquid ingredients first then fold in the solids and stir very lightly before baking. *We never over-process our foods.*

We package our products using special materials to preserve the contents naturally. No artificial preservatives are added, so the shelf-life for our products is not as lengthy as that of highly processed shelf-stable foods. Those foods last for years while Smart for Life foods are one step away from fresh.

When you select the foods you are going to put in your mouth, your body, your body's cells, why not choose the most nutritious, most natural foods you can? I mean organic foods. Organic foods by law must meet federal standards that include restrictions in the use of chemical fertilizers, pesticides, additives, and artificial ingredients. Under current laws, organic foods cannot include use of genetically modified organisms or GMOs.

The use of GMOs in agriculture is a relatively new trend based on the latest techniques in genetics and molecular biology. GMOs were created to elicit high crop yields by using designer seeds that contain pesticides. This is a very unhealthy and dangerous trend, one that has been outlawed in some countries. Potential problems associated with GMOs in crops include allergies, unknown health risks, and threats to the environment and biodiversity.

The inclusion of GMOs is not identified on food labels, so the European Union has regulated against importing foods from the US that may contain GMOs. At this point, most of the American corn supply and much of our soybean supply has been genetically modified. Choosing organic foods is one way of avoiding GMOs.

Smart for Life foods and beverages are made without GMOs. Our products are 60% organic. Our products would be 100% organic but some of our functional ingredients are not available in organic form. However, we include these functional foods in our products because they are essential to appetite suppression and serve to enhance overall health.

Organic foods are more expensive than the non-organic choices. But price is a matter of supply and demand. Once the American public demands more organic foods—and we are doing so; the trend is moving rapidly in that direction—the prices will fall accordingly.

In the meantime, if you just can't afford organic foods or have no access to them, don't worry. Try to buy locally grown foods instead. Visit local produce farms and farmer's markets. Check out your city's community garden, if you have one in your area, and be sure to eat Smart Foods and Superfoods.

If you stay away from the Wrong Foods, you should notice you are spending less money on food overall. Organic foods are costly but so are fast foods and convenience foods. Eating Smart saves you money because you aren't wasting food dollars over-eating junk foods. Even if your food is not all-natural and 100% organic, your Smart for Life diet will be a healthy one, an affordable way to eat that allows for steady weight loss.

Here's a story about a Smart for Life couple who lost weight together, switching to Smart Foods and avoiding the Wrong ones.

Alan and Jenny

Alan and Jenny were married in 2006. A muscular nightclub bouncer, Alan weighed 225 pounds and had very little body fat. His bride was a size 8. But their happy marriage included lots of delicious meals. Jenny was a great cook. They liked hanging out together, often on the couch. With snacks.

They were eating the Wrong Foods.

Within a year of the wedding, Alan weighed 276 pounds. His waist had ballooned from a size 32 to a size 42, and Jenny was wearing a size 14 dress. "We had gotten to the point where we didn't want to go and hang out with people," Alan says. "We didn't feel good about it. We didn't want to be the fat couple in the crowd."

When Alan saw a video of himself dancing around the house with his kids, he was horrified. He looked sweaty and swollen, and his clothes didn't fit right. "I have two young children, and it was extremely difficult for me to keep up and truly enjoy them," he remembers. He was only 32 years old.

Alan wanted to lose the weight and get back in shape. But, due to his 70 hour a week job, he needed a diet plan that would not require a lot of special food preparation or time in the gym. He heard about Smart for Life and decided to sign on. The program didn't require a lot of work in the kitchen, and an exercise program was not mandatory. He found that he liked the food and began to develop a taste for Smart

Foods, including vegetables.

Alan avoided the Wrong Foods and stayed on the diet. He dropped to 205 pounds in less than 6 months.

In the meantime, Jenny got motivated, too. "I didn't want to be known as his fat wife," she says. So she went on the Smart for Life diet herself. She made delicious meals from Smart Foods, and stopped serving Wrong Foods at meals and as snacks.

Jenny lost 60 pounds. She's back in a size 8 dress again.

"When I was so heavy, I would get out of bed in the morning with my feet hurting," Alan recalls. Being uncomfortable was no way to start a 10 hour day spent mostly on his feet. The weight loss changed all that. Losing the weight improved his energy level. His feet stopped hurting. His confidence returned. "Everywhere I go, people that know me recognize my weight loss. This gives me a tremendous boost. Since I lost the weight, my activity and energy have made it possible to enjoy my family. People tell me it looks like I shed 15 years. And now I feel good."

Smart Eating

So now you know what to eat and what not to eat to be Smart for Life. But maybe you'd like some meal and snack suggestions to help you create a kind of daily menu for yourself. No problem. I needed the same kind of assistance when I was first learning how to eat Smart.

In Chapter 6, you'll find a sample week of menus for the RCD as well as recipes for the meals and snacks included, and you'll find a sample week of menus for the Smart Maintenance Diet, for when you've reached your weight goal, plus recipes for those menus, too. I've also included additional recipes for salad dressings, vegetable dishes, healthy snacks, and beverages.

Some people on the program prefer to buy Smart for Life ready-made products and use those for most meals and snacks. You might want to mix up your own cookies or make all your own meals from scratch. These choices are up to you. As long as you eat the Smart Foods and avoid eating the Wrong Foods, you will achieve success on the Smart for Life program.

Smart Breakfasts

The key to a Smart breakfast: avoid eating a high glycemic index meal in favor of a high protein meal. First thing in the morning, everyone—dieters and non-dieters, adults and kids—should eat foods that provide a steady supply of energy so that we can function properly for the entire morning without crashing. We all need to maintain our blood sugar at an efficient level, not too high and not too low. So it is the worst idea possible to gulp down a bowl of processed breakfast cereal. Nobody needs to start the day with a fat-storing sugar-rich meal.

I like to make an egg white omelet with chopped tomato and kale. Experiment with egg whites and you'll find a wide variety of delicious high protein breakfast dishes. Frittatas made with egg whites and diced veggies are great. Some of my patients like a small bowl of Smart for Life cereal or kashi with soy milk. Others are on the run first thing in the morning so they may grab a handful of fresh almonds and drink a glass of low-fat milk for a fast Superfoods breakfast.

Don't be afraid to have fish and veggies when you get up in the morning. The Japanese people do, and they are some of the healthiest, thinnest, and longest living people in the world.

Smart Lunches

You may be wondering what to eat if you can't have a sandwich every day for lunch. Please! Be creative and think outside the lunch box. Sandwiches are not the only luncheon menu option.

What about grilled fish and veggies, a big fresh salad with olive oil and balsamic vinegar, or steamed tofu and vegetables? Make a wrap using lettuce leaves instead of bread to enclose veggies and sliced chicken. If you prefer a snack style lunch, you might like nuts, a small can of tuna in water, some flaxseed crackers and low-fat cheese, raw veggie sticks like celery or carrots with hummus.

Check out our delicious recipe ideas in Chapter 6.

Smart Snacks

Snacks have a bad rap, but the Smart for Life program is based on snacks because eating small healthy meals and snacks throughout the day will send your body's cells the right message: you are not starving and there is no need to store fat.

As long as the snacks you choose are not Wrong Foods.

All the Smart Foods on the list above make terrific snacks. Snacks need not consist of the traditional chips and dips. Why not try raw veggies and plain yogurt, a small piece of grilled fish, a fresh salad with kale? How about smoked salmon? Eat some raw nuts. Drink a glass of low-fat soy milk.

I'm a big fan of baked zucchini slices. Check out our Smart snack recipes in Chapter 6.

Smart Dinners

On the Smart for Life RCD, your dinner meal will consist of up to 12 ounces of lean protein and up to five servings of vegetables. The amounts of protein and veggies you include for dinner will depend on how much you have eaten throughout the day. You will need to keep track of your intake of protein in ounces and veggies in cups on a day to day basis. Use the Food Diary and Menu Planner in the Appendix to help you organize your meals and snacks.

As for dinner itself, an amazing variety of choices are available to you. Fresh or steamed vegetables are terrific, especially when they are organic and in season. Ask at the local produce market what is best and then buy some even if it is a new vegetable you have never eaten before. Wait until you try steamed jicama. Delicious!

Look for fresh fish. I live in Florida, and we have terrific fresh fish. If you live inland, get some fresh frozen fish instead. Try a species you've never tasted before. Cultivate new flavors. Ever try mussels in tomato sauce? How about conch? Be brave: dare to enjoy fresh food!

Try cooking with tofu, yogurt, soy milk, almond milk, and low-fat cheese. You'll be amazed what a topping of low-fat mozzarella on steamed green beans tastes like. Excellent!

I've included quite a few of my favorite dinner recipes in Chapter 6.

Smart Shopping

When you shop for food, the key is to focus on what you *will* buy and ignore the majority of items in the supermarket, the myriad foods that are not high in nutrient value but are supersized and full of empty calories. My patients find it helps to make a shopping list and stick to it. Try not to get seduced by the attractive packaging on all those over-processed foods that will do nothing but send the wrong messages to your body's fat storage cells.

Instead, you can organize your shopping list in the following manner for easy use on your grocery store expeditions.

Produce: Look for fresh vegetables and buy them daily or as often as you can to ensure freshness. In Europe, veggies are stored at room temperature and eaten the same day. You might want to try this. Salads taste so much better when the greens are room temperature. Be sure to buy green, leafy vegetables including kale, collards, and romaine lettuce. Try fermented veggies like Korean kimchi or German sauerkraut. They are great for digestion. Avoid high glycemic potatoes and sweet potatoes. No fruit juices because they are too high in fructose, but you can include fresh fruits like apples, pears, berries, and pomegranates. Limit yourself and keep the serving sizes small. Dried fruits like mango, dates, and pineapple are a great sweet treat once you reach your goal weight. But keep in mind the fact that all fruit is high in fructose, which can send fat-storage messages to your body's cells.

Protein: Go lean on protein and remember to purchase adequate amounts for your daily 10 to 12 ounce serving. Best choices are chicken, fish and other seafood, low-fat milk or soy milk, low-fat yogurt and cheese, and eggs. (You will cook with only the whites, though, as egg yolk is too rich in cholesterol. Dilute the yolks in water and feed to your plants. The nutrients will help them flourish). You may purchase unroasted, unsalted almonds and other raw nuts as well. Tuna and chicken canned in water are okay for occasional quick meals as are the natural, low-sodium deli chicken and turkey made without preservatives. Smoked salmon is good once in a while, too. Experiment with legumes—beans, peas, lentils, tofu, and hummus. Also, you can buy protein powders (like soy, whey, or hemp) made without added ingredients; add the powder to your shakes and smoothies. Or try Smart for Life protein shakes.

These foods are your staples. You will eat a majority of your meals and snacks in the form of vegetables and lean protein.

Grains: Unfortunately, most grains are carbohydrate rich and will spike blood sugar levels rapidly and sharply. Cereals, breads, rice, and pastas tend to have a high glycemic index and do not send good messages to your body's cells. Some exceptions are the Smart for Life high-protein cereals, muesli, rolled oats, kashi, and Kay's Naturals cereals. An occasional bowl of rolled oats or a sprinkle of high protein cereal in yogurt or on a salad is fine, but it is best to minimize grains while you are retraining your body's metabolism.

Beverages: Avoid soft drinks unless they are natural beverages sweetened with stevia. Bottled water is a massive waste of plastic and harmful to the environment. Install a filter in your home and filter your water. Drink your 64 ounces plain, in tea or coffee, or over ice.

Snack foods: You can avoid these aisles entirely. There is nothing in the crowded rows of brightly packaged snack items that can help you to become healthy and trim. Chips, popcorn, packaged foods like sugar-rich cookies, cakes, and other such items will ruin your weight loss efforts and contribute to elevated blood glucose, blood pressure, and blood cholesterol. These foods send the worst possible messages to your body's cells. If you want a healthy crunchy snack, bake thinly sliced veggies and sprinkle with sea salt. Check our healthy snack recipes in Chapter 6. You might want to try Smart for Life organic cookies and other snacks. Remember, the best way to shop Smart is to avoid completely the snack food aisles.

Be sure to buy as much organic food as you can find and afford. Buy locally grown and produced foods, which are fresher and have a lower impact on the environment because they are not trucked across the country to your supermarket. Be sure to read food labels and look for the most natural, least processed foods you can find.

My patients tell me they feel better almost immediately once they begin to eat Smart, and they save money by eliminating sodas, chips, cake mixes, microwavable foods, and other such expenses.

Smart Dining Out

When you are eating Smart for Life, dining out is a pleasure and a treat. But at first, it's a major challenge because the Wrong Foods are all around you, and everyone else is indulging in them. You have to be on guard, and, just like when you enter a supermarket, it is best to plan ahead before dining out.

The following tips seem to really help my patients when they dine out. Memorize this list and then challenge yourself to dine out while remaining Smart. Soon enough, eating Smart in restaurants will become second nature to you, and you'll find the experience even more pleasurable than when you were overindulging—and feeling sorry afterward for over-eating.

Tip #1: Make a plan. Decide in advance what you will order. Find out what restaurant you are going to and what's on the menu. You can usually find fish, seafood, chicken, and salads on menus these days. If there is nothing lean on the menu, ask if the chef can prepare something for you. Restaurants get such requests all the time and are usually happy to fulfill them.

Tip #2: No bread on the table. Just ask them not to bring out the bread basket or to remove it. If you are with a group, pass the bread down to the far end of the table.

Tip #3: Avoid the appetizers or order one as your main meal if it consists of plain vegetables or lean protein. For example, shrimp cocktail can be a Smart choice.

Tip #4: Your protein choice should be baked or grilled, poached or broiled but never fried. Ask your server about the size of the protein serving you are ordering. If it is too large, cut it in half when you are served. Then bag the extra and bring it home with you for another day's meal.

Tip #5: No sauces on your meat, chicken, fish. No buttery, oily toppings on vegetables. No dressing on the salad. Ask for oil and vinegar on the side.

Tip #6: Skip dessert. Or, if you are on the Smart Maintenance diet, split a dessert with the rest of your group. Have a bite or two and that's it. Indulge your sweet tooth, enjoy your splurge, and remain in control. No doggie bag for the leftover dessert.

Tip #7: No alcohol. It is too easy to overdo on drinks and then find your self-control has slipped, and you are overindulging on food as well. Avoid all alcohol while you are on the RCD. On the Smart

Maintenance diet, a glass of red wine is allowed. Red wine is rich in antioxidants, and a regular moderate intake has been linked to good health and longevity. But keep your intake moderate. One glass of a nice red wine is plenty.

If you are in a Chinese or other Asian food restaurant, avoid the white rice in favor of steamed vegetables with chicken or seafood. In Mexican restaurants, try the fajitas and avoid the tortillas in favor of grilled veggies with chicken or seafood. At an Italian restaurant, select a baked seafood dish or a nice chicken dish but not served over pasta. And no pizza—not if you want to eat Smart.

As you move on to the Smart Maintenance diet, you will find that your body's efficient metabolism is able to handle an occasional indulgence. But once you are Smart for Life, your desire to indulge will only be that: occasional.

Restocking Your Pantry

Use all of the supermarket shopping tips provided above to restock your pantry and make your kitchen as Smart as possible. Avoid the urge to fill your shelves with foods you are not going to eat anymore. Stop buying the Wrong Foods. Select only the Smart Foods, and make that the focus of your home menus. Your family might complain at first, but later they will thank you for your attention to their health and weight. Everybody will get healthy, feel better, and become Smart for Life.

If others bring home doggie bags or packaged foods, remember to use personalized stick-on labels to remind yourself not to eat the Wrong Foods. This takes willpower, but soon enough your craving for such foods will diminish. Believe me, if I can give up Oreos and chocolate-covered almonds and *not hear them calling to me anymore*, this will happen to you, too. The longer you remain Smart, the easier resisting unhealthy foods will become.

So, now you know what to eat and what to avoid eating while on your way to a new, healthier weight. I tell my patients to take the Smart Foods list and the Superfoods list and post them in the kitchen somewhere, on a wall or on the fridge. You can post the Wrong Foods list, too, but there is probably no need. *If a food is not on the Smart Foods list, don't eat it.*

Before we move on to the non-dietary components of Smart for Life, here's a story you might find inspiring. Lydia E. is an amazing woman.

Lydia E.

When Lydia E. was 26 years old, she was diagnosed with cancer, underwent a radical hysterectomy, and went through early menopause. Over the years, she gained weight and found herself feeling constantly tired. She hid her body from her husband, embarrassed by the weight she had gained.

When Lydia turned 40, she and her husband adopted a child from the foster care system. An accident had caused severe burns to the boy's chest and face. Lydia and her husband nursed the 15-month-old boy back to health. They cared for him 24/7, taking turns in 12 hour shifts. During this stressful period, Lydia ate on the run, grabbing fast foods and junk foods whenever she had a minute to eat. She ate all the Wrong Foods. Not surprisingly, she gained more weight.

Lydia's son healed nicely and adapted to living in his new home. Lydia was thrilled. But she was disgusted with how her body looked. "I was miserable and made it difficult for my husband. I was moody and snapped at him easily, which made me hate myself even more," she recalls.

She had been on and off a variety of weight loss diets. "Over a period of 15 years, I had used almost every diet pill and plan known and had little or no success. This always made me feel like a failure. Nothing worked." She felt tired all the time, so she did not have the energy to begin an exercise program. She felt trapped in her own body.

Then Lydia E. heard about Smart for Life. She checked out the program online and decided to try it. To protect herself against humiliation, she told few people she had embarked on a comprehensive new diet program. "Because of fear that it might not work. I didn't want to be like those people who say they are quitting smoking and don't!"

Lydia knew she needed to get control of her life, beginning with her eating habits. "I felt out of control, very depressed, and I hated myself," she says.

To her utter amazement, Lydia lost 7 pounds in her first week on Smart for Life. "I was surprised at how I actually did not feel hungry all the time like with all the other diets I had tried," she says. "I actually felt better! And the most surprising part of the Smart for Life plan was how easy it was to do. It never feels like you are on a diet."

Almost immediately, Lydia noticed an improvement in her energy level. "I wasn't feeling so tired all the time. I stopped feeling bloated within the first week. And I felt happy, which I hadn't been in a long time." Things were much better at home, and Lydia and her husband returned to an intimacy level they had not enjoyed in years. Because, Lydia says, "My relationship with my husband greatly improved since I was feeling so much better about myself."

Friends and relatives noticed right away that Lydia was looking and feeling better. When she praised the diet she was on, a number of her coworkers signed up for Smart for Life, too. She made sure to ask others to be supportive of her endeavor. She didn't want to offend anyone when she refused offers of rich foods and party fare.

Lydia was pleased with the support she received while on the diet. She also was happy with the support she obtained from the Smart for Life staff. "You begin to realize very quickly that they are really working with you to attain your goal. After years of searching, I had finally found the program that actually does what it claims to do."

In only 17 weeks, Lydia reached her goal weight. She had lost 45 pounds.

"*You lost lots of weight. How did you do it?* is the question everyone asks me," Lydia E. says now. She credits the Smart for Life diet with not only helping her to shed the weight but giving her the energy she needed to be able to stick to a new way of eating. "I no longer feel tired after supper. I have enough energy to go all day and all evening long. Now I can enjoy working, doing all the household chores, and running after a 2 year old, and I still have energy. Which is amazing! I have my life back."

Part II: Smart Living

"Persistence is the twin sister of excellence. One is a matter of quality; the other a matter of time."

—Marabel Morgan

"Don't ever give up on something or somebody you can't go a full day without thinking about."

—Anonymous

Chapter 4: The Smart for Life Exercise Program

After working as an emergency room doctor, I became the medical director of an executive health program. Our patients included corporate executives and upper level government employees. My patients came to see me for regular checkups or with illnesses and medical issues. Most of these patients were powerful and wealthy. The elite. The opposite of my inner city patients in the ER.

Almost immediately, I noticed something surprising. I could see how, in some ways, the executives were similar to the low income patients I had been treating for years: the high income people were fat, too. Many were obese. And they had the same diet- and weight-related disorders: heart disease, type 2 diabetes, insulin resistance, hormonal problems.

An important component of the executive health program was the weight loss clinic. Because I was responsible for the entire health program, I wanted to make the weight loss clinic as effective as possible. I could see a need for a serious program, so I began to do some research on diets. I wanted to find out whether there were any medically supervised weight loss programs with documented success.

I was determined to help my patients lose weight, and I was still hopeful I might find a plan that worked for me, too.

It seemed like a smart idea to go right to the top, so I looked into the highly regarded medical weight loss programs offered at the best universities in America. I studied the programs being conducted at Harvard, Yale, and Stanford. I also looked at all the work being done at the University of Toronto and McGill University in Canada. Then I incorporated the basic diet, exercise, and psychosocial themes from these esteemed university programs into the program I was offering my patients. I tried out some of the weight loss recipes and tips myself, and I did lose some weight. My patients lost weight as well.

However, we all struggled with the same obstacle to significant success: we found it difficult to remain on the diet because we were forced to prepare the foods required while trying to function at work and at home. You had to make the diet foods and bring them with you while you rushed through your hectic life as a busy doctor, executive, secretary, diplomat, or anyone else. The diet was good; the food was fine, but the program itself never lasted. Life kept getting in the way.

Also, as you may remember, I have a sweet tooth. None of the university diets allowed for that. Plus, I was continuously hungry on the diet, so all the desserts I was missing would call to me. I would forget to prepare or bring with me my special diet lunch, or I would be starving and unable to work and would find myself in front of the vending machines with coins in hand. Or I would go off the diet for this treat or that snack, this special meal or that social event. And before I knew it, I was back at my starting weight.

You must understand the position I was in. I was the director of a medical program for some very important people, and I was their doctor. Every day I was telling these high-level executives that they should lose 10 pounds or 30 pounds or 100 pounds. Yet, I was unable to lose weight and keep it off myself.

I felt like a sham.

So I began to research other weight loss programs. I was looking for medically supervised, non-surgical programs with proven track records of success. I was looking for diets that promised to curb your hunger while you lost weight. I was looking for something that had really worked for others on a long-term basis. Wasn't there a program out there that would help my patients—and me?

My research continued for months. I kept on looking through the scientific literature, reading the bestselling diet books, attending weight loss seminars. But I knew that the truth was this: *I was going to have to invent a weight loss program myself.* A weight loss program that really worked for my busy executives. One that would work for my former patients in the inner city hospital. A weight loss program on which any overweight individual could lose weight without going hungry, without having to spend hours in the kitchen preparing special foods. An affordable, practical, convenient weight loss program. Something smart that anyone could do, a healthy program everyone could follow—for life.

I knew that I was going to have to invent a weight loss program that worked for me and then make it available to my patients—and to everyone else who might need it.

Why Not Exercise the Weight Off?

As you may recall, exercise did not help me to lose the weight I needed to lose. In fact, once I was exercising regularly, I found that I had continuously to increase my activity level to keep my weight in check because the running and swimming, biking and karate served to boost my appetite. After exercising, I needed to eat more. I was hungrier than I had been when I wasn't active, and I ate more. All that physical activity, all those hours in the gym, and I didn't lose a single pound.

But, you are thinking, *if Dr. Sass had just stuck to a diet and continued to exercise, he would have lost those extra pounds.*

That's what I believed, too. I blamed myself and my out of control appetite for my continuous lack of success. But then I did a lot of very careful research, and I found out that everything I had believed about the role of exercise in weight loss was wrong.

The facts are simple: physical activity increases your appetite. The human body is hardwired to signal the appetite center in the brain after energy has been expended, informing you that you need to replenish the energy you have used. Unfortunately, the appetite control mechanisms in the brain do not take into account all those fat stores we might have at the ready. So, after you swim or work out or go for a run, your body tells you to eat. And, if you're like me, you respond to those hunger signals because that's what we are hardwired to do.

But if we have already stored up too much energy in reserve as body fat, we don't really need to eat that much after we exercise. Our fat stores can supply the energy we need. But try telling that to the appetite center in your brain. I know for a fact this doesn't work.

Knowing the facts on exercise and appetite, it might not sound so strange to you that on the Smart for Life program you are told NOT to begin an exercise program. And those who already work out regularly are advised NOT to increase the amount of exercise they are doing while following the Smart for Life weight loss program. This advice, however, is unusual in the weight loss business. Most diet plans come linked to an exercise program: "Start now: join a gym and cut back your food intake." Sound familiar?

It took me a lot of research and years of work with overweight patients to discover what I am sharing with you here: until relatively recently, diet programs included a diet plan and no exercise. *Adding exercise to a weight loss regimen is a relatively recent phenomenon.* And, as anyone who has gone to the local gym lately may testify, exercise for weight loss does not seem to be working for most people. Now you understand why.

A Brief History of Exercise

Until the 1960s, medical researchers and doctors who treated obese patients dismissed the role of exercise in weight loss. In fact, the leading experts advised against exercise, and some prescribed bed rest for those reducing calories significantly. The experts knew that humans burn relatively few calories while exercising and are apt to overeat upon completion of the activity due to a sharp increase in appetite. For example, a 250 pound person would only burn around 200 calories bike riding for 30 minutes while drinking a large soda or eating a commercial protein bar afterward could easily replace those calories and possibly more.

However, during the 1960s, American nutritionists who studied obese rats found that those forced to run on treadmills were leaner than their sedentary peers. At the time, running as a sport had begun to garner national attention. Fitness became a national priority when President Kennedy launched a program in the public schools. The media announced that we needed to get active; there seemed to be a link with our body weight. The "eat less, exercise more" mantra was created.

Unfortunately, the sentiment itself is wrong. Study after study has shown that dieters who exercise vigorously fail to lose weight. Like me, they may get fit, feel better, build muscle, even find that they love to exercise. I still exercise almost daily because I discovered how good it makes me feel, but I do not exercise to lose weight, and I don't advise my patients to do so, either.

Exercise can significantly improve your fitness level. And this is important. It's terrific for your overall health and may increase your longevity. Being physically fit makes you look and feel better. But exercise is not the way to shed pounds.

Smart for Life and the RCD will help you lose weight, not an exercise regimen. You can think of it this way: exercise is for fitness; a healthy weight loss diet is for fatness. And, once you reach your weight goal, exercise is essential for maintaining a healthy weight.

Sometimes it is not possible to exercise for health reasons. Some obese people are unable to exercise. Even taking brief walks would be impossible for them. Some people find they need to lose weight after an accident or illness has forced a period of sedentary living. This does not mean weight loss is not possible. In fact, *a weight loss program works best when you do not increase your physical activity.*

Read the following story of a middle-aged man who could not exercise at all. That is, not until he adopted the Smart for Life program to help him lose weight.

Jim G.

When Jim G. was 55 years old, he was in a bad car accident. He underwent a number of surgeries and began taking prescribed medications, including prednisone, which causes weight gain. He was unable to walk, and he began to add on the pounds. Rapidly.

As his weight ballooned, Jim's health deteriorated: he suffered from sleep apnea and congestive heart failure. He was sick and frightened. The significant weight gain was causing life threatening health issues.

For the next three years, Jim tried a number of weight loss diets. All were unsuccessful. He could no longer tie his own shoes. He couldn't horse around with his grandchildren. He was so disabled that he could not exercise at all. In fact, he was unable to walk more than a hundred feet.

Desperate and scared, Jim went on his computer and surfed the Internet, looking for a diet that might work for him. "After researching several diets, I chose Smart for Life. It made the most sense to me," he wrote to me from his home in Texas.

As he lost weight, Jim found that he could move better. He began to walk a little more each day but not enough to boost his appetite too much. He soon found he was losing 15 to 18 pounds a month "by following this unbelievably easy diet."

After a year on the Smart for Life program, he had lost an incredible 119 pounds. Jim's life turned around.

"My congestive heart disease and sleep apnea have all but disappeared. Breathing is much easier, and I am thinking much more clearly," he reports. "I can tie my shoe laces, walk three miles a day, and play with my grandkids. Life is so much easier now. And fun."

Jim admits he doesn't always eat Smart. "I actually cheat," he says, "and eat whatever I want on special occasions. But I always get back on track without any problems."

Jim G. told me that his health has "vastly improved," and he is happy with reaching his goal weight. "I still struggle with bad eating habits. So I go back to eating Smart for Life cookies when I gain too much weight. It's easy to get right back on the diet."

His family is proud and amazed at his success. Jim is, too: "Unbelievable is all I can say."

Slow and Steady

Like Jim G., my patients find they lose weight steadily if they stick to the program and moderate their physical activity. Patients who are working out several times a week, swimming or jogging every other day, typically choose to continue on their exercise program. This is fine. Everyone else on the Smart for Life program is advised to adopt the RCD and remain on it until reaching their healthy weight goal *while finding subtle ways to be more physically active.*

And when I say subtle, I mean subtle. I do not mean rigorous, or you'll feel hungry and then you'll eat. And if you are like me, you'll go for the Wrong Foods or you'll simply eat too much. And this is not what you want to do while you are on the RCD.

The following activities may be incorporated into your day to subtly improve your fitness and your health without triggering your appetite:

*park your car at the far end of the parking lot and walk to your destination *get off the bus or subway one stop early and walk the extra blocks

*use the stairs instead of the elevator (unless your destination is on the 12th floor—or higher)

*buy small weights and create an upper arm exercise regimen that lasts 5 to 10 minutes

*incorporate stretching exercises into your work day to relieve stress for a few minutes

* get up from the couch and do stretching exercises while you watch the news on TV

*take the dog for a walk once or twice a day

*take the baby out for a walk in the stroller

*walk around outside to get fresh air and sun for 5 to 10 minutes a day

*take a short nature walk whenever you have a chance—at the beach, in a local park, or in your neighborhood—and look at the sky, the birds and other animals, the trees and flowers, the natural beauty around you

*plant and tend a vegetable garden or add some new flowers to your yard

*sign up for a beginner's yoga class

*clean the house, wash the car, wash the windows, rake leaves

*play with the kids: ball, tag, catch, anything fun

*play golf, go bowling, ride your bike for 10 minutes, play a little, enjoy yourself

My patients tell me that eating Smart saves them the time they once spent in fast food lines, preparing big meals, or dining on supersized foods. If you allot an hour for a meal and eating it takes you only twenty minutes, you have another forty you can spend doing something else like walking outside in the fresh air, gardening, or doing yoga.

Adding in Activity

If you find that you are becoming too hungry, the first thing to do is cut back on your physical activities. You might want to keep a record of your activities over a period of time. See if you notice a link between any of your activities and increased eating behaviors.

Remember: there will be plenty of time to exercise once you lose the weight you need to lose. In fact, once you attain your healthy weight goal, the time will be right for adding exercise.

When you reach your desired weight, exercise is mandatory. An exercise program is required to avoid regaining all the lost pounds. Regular exercise is an important aspect of being Smart for Life because to be Smart for Life, you must also be physically active for the rest of your life. Being fit is a major factor in maintaining a healthy body weight, and regular daily activity is essential to efficient body metabolism.

Once you are at your desired weight, you will shift over from the RCD to the Smart Maintenance diet plan. At this point, I tell my patients who are not already exercising regularly that it is time slowly, carefully to add some exercise to their daily routine. This is a balancing act because you don't want to trigger your appetite and then find you are eating too much. You'll need to train yourself to read your own body's signals: is this the right amount of exercise so I will have a good workout without feeling ravenous?

Learning how to balance your food intake with an exercise program takes time. You might want to allow yourself to make a few mistakes. Take it slow. Eventually, you will figure out what works best for you.

If you have adopted some of the subtle activities listed above, the easiest thing to do is simply expand on them. Walk more. Lift weights for 20 or 30 minutes a few times a week. Join a gym. Get on a program with a personal trainer. Bike for half an hour. Start jogging. Take up a sport.

The choice is yours.

Use the Exercise Planner in the Appendix to help you create your own physical activity regimen. Choose some fun activities, the kind of exercise you will want to do often.

My former patients at Smart for Life are different kinds of people with different lifestyles and schedules, but my successful former patients all have one thing in common: they each have a personalized exercise regimen they have created for themselves. Their exercise programs may include only one activity done daily or a variety of physical activities conducted on a regular basis.

Some people walk, others run, and a few of us fly. I'm a big fan of kite boarding, which is like surfing while attached to a huge kite that can lift you above the ocean when the wind is right. I would never have been able to kite board when I was fat! It takes a lot of strength and stamina, which I have built up over the years. Once I lost the excess weight that was holding me back, I was able to select from a wide array of fantastic forms of exercise, and you will be able to do so as well.

But that's later on, once your weight is under control. Right now, I want you to keep exercise in mind, but not focus on it. At this time, you'll need to focus your attention and energy on sticking to the RCD and avoiding feeling too hungry so you can remain on the program.

My patient Stan W. is a perfect example of someone who got Smart then fit and saved his life in the process.

Stan W.

Stan W. credits Smart for Life with saving his life.

In 2000, the tax accountant was in a serious car accident and spent months recuperating. His weight climbed steadily until the 6'2" father of two tipped the scales at 362 pounds: "My back was killing me, and I developed sleep apnea."

One day Stan passed out. This freaked him out. His doctor told him he had better lose weight or he was on his way to an early heart attack. Stan was not even 40 years old.

"All of my physicians had told me to lose weight, but none of them had any real-life answers as to how to accomplish that," he recalls. So Stan began to look for a diet plan he might be able to follow, one that did not require exercise because he was in no shape for that. Not yet.

When Stan heard about the Smart for Life program, it sounded like a good fit. He didn't want to mess with anything complicated, and he was not able to exercise. The program seemed like something he might be able to follow for a while. After all, he had more than 100 pounds to lose.

To his surprise, the program worked. Stan never felt hungry, and he found the diet easy to follow. His wife helped him to eat right by being supportive and encouraging, and he began feeling more energetic. The additional support he received from the Smart for Life staff helped him ride out some slow times when his weight seemed to plateau.

Over the course of six months, Stan lost 95 pounds. After a year, he was down 122. Now he has reached his goal weight with a total loss of 142 pounds. And he's added in a regular program of exercise.

"I started working out, and now I feel more healthy than I ever have in my entire life. My health problems, including the sleep apnea, have disappeared," Stan told me. "Even my wife notices the difference in my energy level. Our love life is better than ever!"

Stan does find that his weight fluctuates. Sometimes he is "casual" with his food choices over the weekends. He has also increased his workout schedule to accommodate karate classes 3 or 4 times a week in addition to going to the gym every other day. He has added considerable muscle to his frame, and he is currently working on his Green Belt.

However, all that exercise makes it hard for Stan not to overeat. "I find myself very hungry at night," he admits. "I get home from a workout, and I want to eat." He tries to manage his hunger with Smart for Life products like the cookies and shakes. At this point, Stan is still learning how to balance the physical activity he loves with his body's need for food so he can maintain his desired weight for life.

Stan W. is much stronger now than he was before Smart for Life, and he's much more fit. "If you asked me in 2008 if I could see myself doing what I do (and can do) now, I would have said I couldn't," he admits with pride.

Sometimes physical hunger is not the culprit when we go off a weight loss plan. I know from experience—my own and that of my patients—that over-eating is not always in response to physical hunger. We'll eat the Wrong Foods because they are there. It's a celebration or a holiday. Someone we love is urging us to eat. We're out to dinner, and everything Wrong is calling to us, or we feel like we just cannot help ourselves; we're craving something Wrong, Wrong, Wrong.

Staying motivated to stick to the Smart for Life program is essential to long-term weight loss success. And staying on track is a challenge. Believe me, I know. There are situations and people in our lives who will sabotage our weight loss efforts. Some of us must deal with serious food addictions. Getting and staying fit is not easy. The challenges are real.

I'm going to discuss all this in the next chapter. But first, you might like to read a story about someone who faced some of these challenges and chose to be Smart. In fact, this young man saved his health and his career by becoming Smart for Life.

Mitch B.

A big guy with a muscular build, Mitch B. is an athlete. He's 6'2" tall and works out every day. He's built. You wouldn't want to mess with him.

Mitch B. had never had a weight problem. Staying fit was an integral part of his lifestyle, and he didn't worry about what he ate. He didn't think he needed to. But then his doctor told him he had type 2 diabetes. Mitch was shocked. He didn't feel sick, but the symptoms had been subtle. The test results were unequivocal: he had diabetes.

His doctor prescribed insulin medication. The drug made Mitch gain weight. For the first time in his life, he got fat. His belly protruded, and, before he knew it, Mitch B. weighed over 300 pounds.

A nationally known corporate trainer, Mitch was desperate to improve his appearance. There was no room for fat guys on the dais. No way! His self-confidence, essential to his profession, had started to flag, and his energy wasn't what it needed to be. The excess weight was threatening his career, and wasn't being overweight even worse for his diabetes?

A friend of Mitch's had recently trimmed down. She looked like a million bucks. Mitch complemented her and asked how she had lost so much weight. She told him: Smart for Life.

After his friend explained how easy it was to stay on the Smart for Life diet, Mitch looked up the program online. He liked the sound of the Smart for Life weight loss plan. It seemed like the kind of program that would fit into his lifestyle, which involved significant travel and required consistently high energy. He needed to be sharp. He couldn't be hungry and cranky. He didn't want to have to worry about cooking a lot of meals. He needed a weight loss plan he could take on the go. The food had to taste good, keep him full. And the food couldn't be high in sugar; he wasn't able to eat stuff like that anymore. He needed low glycemic index foods in his diet.

Smart for Life looked like it would fit the bill.

In fact, Smart for Life worked wonderfully. Mitch lost 58 pounds without feeling hungry or tired. He feels a lot better and looks a lot trimmer. "People do not recognize Mitch now!" says his fiancee. He's fit, and soon he may be able to stop taking insulin.

If Mitch were my patient at a Smart for Life Weight Management Center instead of someone who went on the program over the Internet, I would probably recommend that he wean himself off the insulin entirely. If his blood glucose levels are normal, which I am confident that they are after almost a year on the Smart for Life program, his diabetes is basically cured. As long as he continues to eat Smart, he should be able to keep his blood sugar in the normal range.

Mitch looks fit and strong again. Now when Mitch B. gets up on the dais, he has all the confidence he needs to be a success.

Chapter 5: Staying Smart for Life

Once I realized I would have to design a diet program myself, one that would work for me and for other busy people who struggled with their weight, I became obsessed with the challenge. I read voraciously, combing the medical literature for ideas I might use to create a successful weight loss program. I knew my program would be based on the most reliable medical studies plus cutting edge research in the fields of food science, nutrition, genetics, molecular biology, and psychology.

My research took months. I poured over the available medical literature. I wanted to know why diets fail, how nutrients and food ingredients influence body weight. I wanted to which foods assist in weight loss, and which foods hinder it. I explored the newest and the most obscure scientific research, talked to obesity experts and food scientists, visited food labs and test kitchens.

During my studies, I heard about a doctor who was using a specially designed cookie as a meal replacement. He had been having some success with his program. This intrigued me. So I contacted him and tested out his diet plan.

I did not like the taste of the little cookies. Plus, there were preservatives I preferred not to include in my diet. However, I liked having something quick and simple to eat whenever I felt hungry. The cookies calmed my sweet tooth, so I didn't crave desserts. I could eat on the run and not feel terribly hungry.

After 2 weeks, I had lost 10 pounds. And that impressed me. My pants were loose, and I felt good. I had energy, I wasn't starving, and I felt like I could remain on the program longer, maybe even long enough to lose the weight I needed to lose.

I was hooked.

One thing bothered me, though. I wanted to eat organic, natural foods. These cookies had a lot of artificial ingredients. I couldn't see eating them for any significant period of time. They seemed, finally, unhealthy to me.

However, I was so impressed with my own success that I recommended the cookies to my patients. They loved them. People were losing weight and praising the convenience of the diet. I decided to visit the doctor who had invented the program.

The doctor welcomed me and seemed open to my suggestions and ideas. He could see the advantages of creating a more natural cookie product. So we decided to work together on his cookies to try to improve them nutritionally.

The cookie diet he was advocating had some very successful aspects but needed to be refined. This was in 2002. People were informed. They wanted to eat healthy, natural foods. Dieters felt the same way. If we were going to ask people to consume our weight loss products daily for months or even years, shouldn't we supply them with the healthiest foods possible? I also believed the cookies needed to be more filling and lower in sugar. Overweight people tend to suffer from insulin resistance. I thought the cookies should help to stabilize blood sugar, not increase it.

My own weight was still 30 pounds over where I wanted it to be. But I couldn't live on the doctor's diet cookies. I needed healthy foods in my day as well. For me, the cookie diet had worked only temporarily. I wanted to create a program that could help with weight loss and weight maintenance *for life.*

The doctor and I didn't agree on everything. That's not unusual in business. But after a while, I had to admit to myself that his cookie diet was not the weight loss program I had been searching for. The flaws were too significant.

Once again, I faced the truth: a new program was required, and I would have to design it myself. Creating the perfect plan was up to me. The other doctor's cookie diet wasn't working for me, not for the long-term. And I knew this particular cookie diet would not help other people to lose weight healthfully and keep it off permanently. I had to face the facts: I still needed to create my own diet program, one based on healthy, natural, easy-to-eat convenience foods that could be eaten throughout the day as small meals and snacks.

Working with food scientists, I began to develop my own special weight loss products. I attended trade shows, spoke to diet food experts, and met with chefs and nutritionists. These professionals provided me with information and ideas for creating the best food products for weight loss. And I hired the best people to work on creating Smart for Life products.

My first product was a 60% organic cookie made without preservatives. I used triple-filtered water in my cookie recipe to make sure the product was as pure as possible. No additives. Only the best ingredients. And it tasted great. Not too sweet but sweet enough to restrain my sweet tooth. Plus, the cookie provided amazing appetite suppression. I had included ingredients specially designed to cut down on hunger, and the cookies really helped to curb my appetite.

After many years of research, I knew a successful weight loss program would include several small meals or snacks throughout the day plus a healthy meal at night. So I substituted my special organic cookies for all of my daytime meals, and my wife provided a nice lean dinner each night, typically a big salad, steamed vegetables, and chicken or fish.

The weight came off quickly, and it kept coming off until I had lost the entire 30 pounds I needed to lose.

Success at last! But I wondered: would my weight loss success last? Was I permanently trim for life?

That was more than ten years ago, so I can tell you this: I have not regained the weight I lost. And I never will. My body is metabolically efficient, I feel good, and I look like a physician who practices what he preaches, a doctor who has created a weight loss program that really works—for him as well as his patients.

Now, don't get me wrong: I still gain weight sometimes. Holidays are tough: lots of good food around, calling to me. Over the holidays, I may just respond to the call of pumpkin pie and roast duck! So I usually gain 5 or 6 pounds over Thanksgiving and Christmas, but then I return to the Smart for Life weight loss program, and, by February, I am back to my goal weight—what is now my normal weight.

I'm not fat anymore. If you saw me on the street now, you would say I am trim. That makes me happy.

To maintain my weight, I exercise regularly, and I eat my own cookies throughout the day on weekdays while I'm busy at work. On the weekends, I will eat other foods during the day. I like egg-white omelets for breakfast and nice dinners at home or in a restaurant. Sometimes I even have dessert.

But on Mondays, I go back to eating Smart for Life cookies again because it took me years to lose those 40 pounds. It took years of suffering, starving, sweating, and striving—until I created Smart for Life and got lean and Smart—for life.

Staying on the Smart Path

When you are following the Smart for Life program, you will not feel like you are dieting because you are eating healthy foods in generous amounts, so you should not be hungry or deprived. And you are retraining your mind along with your body by supplying your cells with the right messages about food energy, nutrition, and health. So, as you lose the weight you need to lose, you are actively relearning how to eat. And that is the point of Smart for Life: to learn how to eat to lose weight *and remain fit and healthy for the long-term.*

As time passes, it will become easier for you to eat Smart and thus stay fit and lean. Nothing tastes as good as thin feels. Once you know how great it feels to be in shape, then you'll become determined to stay that way. I'm a living example of this. So are many of my former patients. We never want to be fat again. Never!

But we will be the first to admit that it is not an easy journey. There are many challenging obstacles to permanent weight loss and healthy living. The most common roadblocks include

*social food obsessions—friends and relatives who would willingly or unwittingly sabotage our weight loss efforts

*food addictions—some of us must avoid those foods that trigger compulsive over-eating

*weight gain danger zones—holidays, birthdays, and special events can wreak diet havoc

*lack of support—family, friends, and other sources of moral support are key to success

*the food industry—modern food corporations have a major role in the current obesity epidemic, and their products and advertisements have a significant influence on our health

Fortunately, there are Smart ways to minimize the obstacles on your journey to healthy, permanent weight loss success. I'll share the facts and tips I provide my patients at Smart for Life Weight Management Centers with you here.

After that, it's up to you to make Smart choices. You'll be the one who has to weigh the consequences of your actions. And, if you want to be lean and fit, you'll be Smart. You'll choose the Smart thing to do every time.

Or almost every time, and that will be enough.

Patient X

One of the most interesting and memorable patients at my Smart for Life Weight Management Center in Boca Raton, Florida, was a very attractive, well-to-do woman in her late 40s. Let's call her Miss X.

Miss X pulled into the parking lot in a new Mercedes. She wore expensive clothing and fashionable shoes, and her hair and nails were impeccable. She was highly educated and had an executive position in a local company. In every way, Miss X appeared to be a success.

However, when I met with her for the first time in my office, Miss X told me she had a serious issue with maintaining her weight. At the time, she was somewhat overweight. She had around 30 pounds she needed to lose. But her main problem was a pattern of weight gain, loss, and regain.

Miss X informed me she gained 40 to 50 pounds every couple of years. She would go on a diet, lose some of the weight, maybe 20 to 30 pounds, only to regain all the lost weight. And then she would gain more. This pattern had plagued her all of her adult life.

Miss X had tried every diet she'd ever read about. She had been to diet doctors; she had joined gyms. Most programs worked temporarily, but she remained locked into the cyclical pattern. Because she was almost 50 years old, she was concerned because the weight was getting harder and harder to lose.

When I asked Miss X if she knew why she seemed to be trapped in this repetitive weight cycle, she surprised me with an intriguing story. "When I was a child," she recalled, "my mother was kind of a hippie. She only prepared natural foods that were vegetarian and very healthy. Vegetables, fruits, whole-grain breads and cereals—these were the only kinds of foods we had in the house."

A diet like that should have set Miss X up for a lifetime of healthy eating. However, this was not the case. The truth is far stranger.

During her youth, Miss X's grandmother lived with her and her mother. The grandmother was old-fashioned, and she did not approve of the natural diet being served. "My grandmother was worried that I wasn't getting proper nutrition. She thought I would not grow well, that I needed a more all-American diet to be healthy and reach my potential," Miss X explained. But the grandmother could not convince Miss X's mother to feed the child differently. So the grandmother decided to do something herself about what she regarded as her granddaughter's deficient diet.

Miss X's grandmother was not honest with Miss X's mother. Behind her back, the grandmother would go to the supermarket and buy what she thought of as "good food" for a growing child. Then she would wait until Miss X was alone, usually in the bathtub.

Miss X remembered how her grandmother would suddenly appear in the bathroom with a "treat" in hand. While little Miss X took her bath, her grandmother would feed her cold-cuts, sliced meats and cheeses, high calorie snacks and desserts. Miss X was told that the nightly visit was their little secret, so she did not tell her mother what was going on. Miss X was too young to understand anyway, and to her the visits with special foods became "normal."

Miss X put on weight. Her mother was perplexed and did not understand why her daughter was pudgy. Miss X didn't really understand it herself at the time, and the grandmother thought the weight gain was good, a healthy change for the little girl.

In this way, the sneaky food game continued for years, and Miss X's mother never found out what was going on behind her back.

As Miss X got older, the game was modified. "When I was in my teens, my grandmother would hide candy bars under my pillow. Of course, I ate them. It was a sign of her love for me. How could I refuse?" Miss X explained to me. And, during meal times, Miss X ate the natural foods her mom had so lovingly prepared.

Miss X was pleasing both of the women who loved her by eating what they each provided for her. She grew up eating too much and feeling confused about her relationship with food.

"I have a love-hate relationship with food," Miss X admitted to me. No surprise there. Miss X told me she had worked with a psychiatrist, a psychologist, and other specialists on her food issues, but she continued to struggle with her weight.

When she came to Smart for Life, Miss X was committed to losing the excess weight once and for all. She was tired of her emotional cycle and the toll it was taking on her body and psyche. She had a good understanding of the underlying issues that contributed to her weight problem. She was willing to try anything.

I advised her to try our Fixed Meal Plan. This Smart for Life diet plan is very rigid and controlled. I recommend it only for those patients who are dealing with food addictions or other psychological issues relating to food compulsions. Usually, after a few weeks on the Fixed Meal Plan, weight is lost, hunger is under control, and the patient can gradually add other foods to their daily intake. More on the Fixed Meal Plan, including menus and recipes, in Chapter 6.

I thought Miss X would prefer the Fixed Meal Plan because that way she would not have to think about the foods she was eating. Every meal was planned for her. She would not have to choose between her mother's natural foods and her grandmother's treats. Instead, Miss X was able to focus on what was best for her body, and she could silence those two old but influential voices in her head.

Miss X lost the 30 pounds she needed to shed. She was thrilled. When she reached her weight goal, she told me she was sure this time she was done with her weight struggle. She looked fantastic as she hopped in her Mercedes and drove off under the perfect Florida sky.

Unfortunately, once she left the program, I lost track of her, so I don't know if Miss X has been successful in keeping off the weight roller coaster caused by her highly unusual upbringing. I can only imagine that, if she needed help, Miss X would come see me again, so I imagine her as I saw her that last day, trim and fit and happy.

Social Food Obsessions

We are a culture addicted to gastroporn. Cooking shows, alluring new food trends, dazzling restaurants, and celebrity chefs dominate the media and serve as a focus of public attention. It seems cool, hip, trendy, and luxurious to eat excessive and unhealthy food. We've become obsessed with food.

When humans are well fed, our interest in food should decline. Typically, starving people—including those on restrictive and unfulfilling diets—are obsessed with food while everyone else eats adequately and gets on with the rest of life. This does not seem to be the case with our modern-day, well-fed populace. Even though we have plenty to eat, we seem to have become more and more infatuated with food.

Our obsession means food has become the central focus of nearly all social events, and these food-dominated events occur regularly, even daily, and there is no escaping the feasts and tempting foods.

The endless series of birthday parties in schools, for example, means that each kid in a class brings in cake and goodies on his or her special day. This can result in as many as 30 birthday parties a year every year for your kids, beginning at age 4 or 5. College dorms are notorious for pizza nights, not to mention keg parties with lots of snack foods. Then the beat goes on for sports events, poker nights, and weekends in general. No office birthday, promotion, or other special day can pass without a cake, drinks, and lots of socializing around the food table.

It is almost impossible to avoid food, unhealthy food, in today's food-obsessed culture. It seems that these days, wherever there is enough food, there is really too much food—and certainly too much of the Wrong Foods.

I think the reasons for our current social food obsession include the following:

*many overweight people are on (and off and on again) weight loss diets that do not satisfy their needs, resulting in food fantasies and obsessions

*widespread nutritional deficiencies due to poor eating habits and over-processed foods make us prone to food obsessions for physiological reasons because our bodies crave the nutrients we are not obtaining from what we eat

*insulin resistance and fluctuating blood sugar levels, now common due to overweight and poor eating habits, are making us feel hungry more often, so that we think more about food

*typically huge portion sizes in packaged foods and restaurant meals mean we tend to eat more and thus believe we want/need more food

*massive and constant advertising of unhealthy foods places thoughts and images of eating in our minds continuously throughout the day

All of the above can make eating healthy foods in proper, adequate amounts a difficult task. Although it is natural to consume what your body needs when you are hungry and to stop eating when you have taken in an appropriate amount of food energy, we have forgotten how to do this. Instead, eating for good health has become a challenge in the face of continuous occasions that offer the opportunity to overindulge. Plus, everyone else around us appears to be over-eating and, in many instances, encouraging us to join in.

When my patients embark on the Smart for Life program, I warn them that they will have to be strong willed. They will have to say no and sometimes seek ways to avoid social events built around overindulging. This is a huge challenge. But it can be done. You know the saying "Please, Universe, if you can't make me thin, make all my friends fat."

Here are my tips for avoiding social indulgences and sabotage:

Tip #1: Plan ahead. Bring your Smart Foods with you to social events or learn the menu in advance so you know what you will be eating.

Tip #2: Don't attend social events when you are hungry. Have a snack beforehand so you won't be ravenous when you arrive and vulnerable to temptation.

Tip #3: Try to situate yourself at social events so you are not near the food. Stand across the room, away from the party platters. Get yourself a cup of ice water and carry it with you so that your hands are full.

Tip #4: Don't drink alcohol. If you let your guard down with a few drinks, you may find yourself diving into the party fare with abandon.

Tip #5: Ask friends and family to be supportive of your weight loss journey. Explain the Smart for Life program and ask those close to you to avoid buying foods that are not on your diet or encouraging you to indulge in the Wrong Foods.

Tip #6: If someone seems to be sabotaging your weight loss efforts, avoid that person as much as possible. If need be, confront the person and ask him or her to stop interfering. Sometimes people feel uncomfortable when others change and are unaware that they are being difficult.

Tip #7: Don't watch all those cooking shows on television! Channel surf through the food advertisements. They're annoying anyway. In fact, the less television you watch, the easier it will be to avoid Wrong Foods in favor of healthy eating.

Tip #8: Find nonfood ways of socializing with others. Take a class, join a book club, find a friend who will take short walks with you. If you hang around people who always seem to eat to socialize, confide in them about your weight loss goals. Once they understand your journey, people are more apt to be supportive.

Tip #9: Form a support group with others who are attempting to lose weight, get fit, or make other life changes. Sometimes just being a supportive friend gives you all the support you need yourself. Remember, you can always contact us at Smart for Life for online or phone support during your weight loss journey.

Food Addiction

Too many of us are obsessed with food and gastronomic pleasures. This is a social and cultural issue. For you as an individual, all the advertisements and inducements might be problematic. Individual change requires focused and diligent effort.

For some, food obsession can evolve into a more serious psychological disorder. If you are so food obsessed that, even when you are not physically hungry, you cannot stop thinking about food—notably the Wrong Foods—then you may be suffering from a food addiction.

Food addiction is a serious, compulsive disorder and may take different forms: starving oneself, eating an excessive amount then vomiting, or simply over-eating. You could have a food addiction if you exhibit the following symptoms:

*you are obsessed with thoughts of food and possibly with the amount of food you eat or do not eat; you gain most of your emotional pleasure from this kind of thinking

*you tend to eat when you are stressed, worried, anxious, sad, or feeling bad about something; you feel worse after eating then eat more

*you feel guilty when you eat

*you play psychological games with food like hiding it, always eating alone, or pretending not to eat

* you avoid food and food-related events to an extreme degree as if you are unable to control yourself around food

*you have a love-hate relationship with food, or you see food as an enemy to be conquered rather than enjoyed

Food addicts may require psychological counseling or medical support during weight loss efforts. It is difficult enough to lose weight when you do not have strong emotional issues around eating, but weight loss may prove impossible if you do. That our brains keep our bodies fat seems like a paradox, but it is an accurate assessment of one of the biggest hurdles to permanent weight loss. That is, you must suffer enough psychologically to become motivated to change, but if you suffer too much emotionally, the struggle may hinder your efforts at change.

Psychological hurdles can seem discouraging, and yet I want you to feel optimistic about the possibility of permanent lifestyle change. I was able to change my eating behaviors, and thousands of individuals who have adopted the Smart for Life program have also been able to rid themselves of unhealthy food issues. Believe me, you *can* change your relationship with food, no matter how entrenched your food addiction may be. You can overcome your obstacles with Smart for Life.

However, let me say this: *The contemporary convenience food diet with all of the added fats and sweeteners, the giant supersized portions, and continuous seductive advertising is making food addicts of us all.*

Over-eating of Wrong foods is a global problem. In places where the people can afford to eat, there is a cultural tendency to overdo on nutritionally empty but widely available foodstuffs. As the economic viability of a society improves, the diet declines, and people develop food-related health issues.

So, please do not feel alone in your struggles with food. The processed food industry is a $500 billion a year business. Scientific research has shown that the over-processed foods that make up the average diet include ingredients *designed* to addict us. Food companies employ psychologists and food scientists who conduct research and laboratory testing to discover exactly which food ingredients will entice us to eat more than we need—and keep coming back for more.

In fact, animal studies with rats have shown that fatty foods like bacon and rich sweets like cheesecake trigger neurochemical responses in the brain that mimic those caused by drugs like heroin and cocaine. Researchers believe a biological reward system in the brain is activated by high fat and sugar rich foods, and that the same reward system responds similarly to the use of addictive drugs. Laboratory studies indicate the overconsumption of fatty junk foods leads to addiction responses in the brain that, in turn, cause compulsive eating.

What does this mean? Eating fast foods and rich desserts causes a kind of pleasurable feeling in us that can easily become addictive and repeated consumption of the Wrong Foods can set up a neurochemical cycle in the brain that causes us to eat and eat, compulsively. It may be as difficult to kick a burger and fries or chocolate habit as it would be to quit crystal meth.

I will admit to being a food addict. As you know, it was very difficult for me to quit grabbing handfuls of chocolate-covered almonds even though I urgently wanted to lose weight. And for years, despite my efforts to drop pounds, all the Wrong Foods kept calling to me until I ate them--until I substituted the Smart for Life cookies. Smart for Life is how I was able to control my own food addiction.

I will not tell you change is easy, because getting new, good habits is not. In fact, you will never be able to *cure* your food addiction or your weight problem. The problem—that is, the food—will always be there. However, *you can control your food addiction and your weight.*

If I can do it and thousands of my patients can do it, so can you.

My patients tell me they find it helps to admit to themselves they are food addicts. The process is the same for alcoholics who successfully control their drinking: admit the problem and seek support. *Hello, I am Dr. Sass, and I am a food addict. I need to rely on Smart for Life to control my obsession with food.*

You might want to approach your food addiction in this time-honored manner. And do seek support. Having a safety net of friends and like-minded colleagues is essential. An addiction, including a food addiction, is very powerful. If you have struggled with food related psychological mine-fields for years, your addiction can have quite a hold on you emotionally and physically.

So please feel free to call us or contact us online. You can find a Smart for Life Weight Management Center near you—or talk to a therapist who specializes in food addictions. Set up a support system for yourself as you move ahead on this challenging journey to achieve and maintain a healthy weight.

For inspiration, read how a young woman with a lifelong food addiction was able to take control and remain in control with Smart for Life.

Brenda M.

She was in a bad relationship and couldn't get out of it. Brenda M. had an unhealthy relationship with food.

"I was 30 years old, overweight, and had never been in a relationship—except with food" is how she describes her food addiction. "I was addicted. I used to consume 5000 calories or more in one sitting without feeling full."

She was acutely lonely, and she felt bad about herself. Brenda knew she needed to make a change in her life. When a local radio disc jockey talked about his weight loss success with Smart for Life, Brenda became interested in the program. She decided to take a chance on love—for herself.

As soon as Brenda began the program, she felt she was regaining a sense of control over herself and her addiction. "The frequent, small portions gave me the discipline I desperately needed," Brenda says. By consuming only Smart Foods, she found her addiction to the Wrong Foods lessening its hold on her. She was finding a way to say good bye to her bad relationship.

She began to change her attitude toward food. She realized she could look at food as a source of energy, nutrition, and satisfaction when she felt hungry rather than as a substitute for her emotional needs. She withdrew from food as a psychological crutch and turned to food as a way to meet her physical needs. Her *real* physical needs rather than her addiction's cravings. Being able to make a distinction between food as nutrition and food as love changed Brenda's life.

As the weeks went by and Brenda lost weight, she developed a new relationship with food. She didn't abandon food for a new lover; she made a pact with food: she would eat what her body needed to be healthy and no more.

Brenda M. remained on the Smart for Life program, and the weight dropped off. "Now I'm 32," she says. "I'm 100 pounds lighter and still using Smart for Life for maintenance. I'm healthier and happier, and I have finally found love. Not only from my boyfriend but for myself."

Weight Gain Danger Zones

Holidays, birthdays, and special events are difficult if you are trying to lose weight. And there are so many of them! Every week another party, special day, dinner out, reason to celebrate. It is indeed a challenge to bypass all the Wrong Foods and still enjoy yourself.

But certain times of the year are almost impossible to get through without gaining a few pounds. My patients struggle with what I call the weight gain danger zones: Halloween, Thanksgiving, and Christmas through New Year's Day.

I must admit: I still gain a small amount of weight every year during the weight gain danger zones. I like to treat myself once a year to some of the holiday foods that are special to me and my family, but then I return to eating Smart again after the first of the year, and by February I'm back to my weight goal, my now normal weight. But believe me, I know how much of a challenge it is to get through those weight gain danger zones intact.

Here are some tips I share with my patients each fall so that they can make it through the end of the year with the least amount of weight gain while still enjoying the holiday spirit:

Tip #1: Plan ahead. Know what's on the menu and decide in

advance what foods you will eat. Eat these foods first so that you are not too hungry. That way you will not fall prey to the lure of the Wrong Foods.

Tip #2: Use a small plate when eating at a buffet. Your meal will look larger and more satisfying to you—and to your hosts.

Tip #3: Allow yourself a glass of red wine or champagne. One glass. And be sure not to overdo, or you may find your willpower has disappeared along with your good judgment.

Tip #4: Do not overindulge! This can be a matter of life and death: many overweight people end up in an Emergency Room after eating and drinking their way there. Eat small amounts, eat slowly, and drink lots of water. You are at risk because you are overweight so BE CAREFUL.

Tip #5: Learn to say "no thank you." This is essential. You do not need to eat everything you are offered. Your hosts will present the food, and it is up to you to select carefully and eat wisely.

Tip #6: Ask friends and family to be supportive. Tell them you are still on the Smart for Life program and will not be eating everything on the menu. Then be firm.

Tip #7: Be active. Get outside and take a walk, play with the kids or grandkids, move around. Hanging around the kitchen or TV room is an invitation to trouble.

What I tell myself as well as my patients is this: try to remain as Smart as possible and eat mostly Smart Foods over the holidays. In between the danger zones, be 100% Smart. That way, you can enjoy a special treat here and there while continuing to eat Smart. Even though it is that challenging holiday time, you can still be sure to serve yourself healthy foods in appropriate amounts, eat only when you are hungry, and feel good about your weight loss progress for the year.

When I was fat, I felt guilty and blamed myself. I knew it was up to me to take control of my food addictions and unhealthy eating behaviors. What I did not realize at the time was this: my overweight condition was not totally my own fault. Living as I did—and still do—in a time of food abundance with convenience foods, fast foods, and unnatural foods available 24/7, my body weight was also under the considerable influence of the modern food industry.

And there was this striking fact: *the food industry was profiting by my over-eating.*

The food industry is profiting from *your* over-eating behaviors, too.

The facts are clear and have been for decades, ever since we decided to industrialize our food supply. Much research has been done and billions of dollars spent to ensure that we buy this brand over that brand and in the largest possible amounts. Food companies want our brand loyalty early, and they want us to purchase often. These corporations do everything they can and spend billions of dollars to make sure we eat and eat and eat because our consumption, our hunger, means that we will buy, buy, buy from them.

To compete with one another for our food dollars, the modern food industry creates products that lead to over-eating and weight gain. Thus, although the food industry is not totally to blame for the current obesity epidemic, the truth is we couldn't have become obese without the major food corporations and their products.

When I say food industry, I'm including the packaged-goods companies, food and beverage corporations, supermarkets, and restaurants. Ever since Swanson invented the first frozen meal, dubbed a "TV dinner" back in 1953, we have been hooked on fast, easy foods. Our desire for tasty and fresh foods was supplanted almost overnight by the widespread acceptance of convenient meals. We became the kind of people who will grab artificial foods on the run, eat in a fast food line, or pop something in the microwave rather than take the time to create a healthy, nutritious meal.

Our willingness to eat junk has proven to be enormously profitable for the food industry—and enormously detrimental to our waistlines not to mention our overall health. Industrialized foods are high in all of the ingredients that contribute to chronic disease and absent or pitifully low in the nutrients we need for good health and longevity.

Federal policies are not helping the situation. It's great that Michelle Obama declared war on childhood obesity. However, the current national food guidelines are not conducive to healthy eating. The newest federal advice has been summarized in the oversimplified "Choose My Plate" icon, a multicolored image of a dinner plate divided into quadrants to indicate equivalent servings of fruits, vegetables, grains, and proteins with a smaller circle to represent a serving of dairy foods. No guidelines are provided regarding portion control, no distinction between the food choices in each category. More than $2 million was spent to create and launch the latest federal nutrition education campaign that will undoubtedly be of little or no help to overweight kids and adults.

To make matters worse, our government subsidizes the industries that are making us fat and unhealthy. Farm bill subsidies contribute to the high cost of fresh produce by deflating the prices of certain products like corn and soy, keeping the processed foods made from them cheap and popular. The food industry invests in products that make the biggest profit, focusing on cheap commodities rather than on higher priced fruits and vegetables. In this way, our federal policies promote low-cost over-processed foods high in unhealthy fats and sugars, supporting unhealthy eating habits and making them economically attractive.

Obviously, we cannot rely on the government to solve our food supply issues. The food industry itself needs to step up to the plate and make some significant changes in the products they sell. With different, healthier ingredients and elimination of the artificial ones, food companies could produce superior products that consumers would buy, buy, buy—without compromising their own and their family's health.

If we can provide health food at Smart for Life, surely the mega-food corporations with all their money, their laboratories, and their test kitchens full of experts could create healthier, better tasting, more nutritious, and natural food products. Until they do, however, consumers must read labels and shop carefully, check over menus, and ask questions. We need to be keenly aware of the food we are eating, how it was prepared, and what ingredients are in it. Smart consumers will select natural foods that are unprocessed or minimally processed.

As consumers, we must demand better foods and spend our food dollars only on the kinds of foods we want to see in the marketplace. Until the food industry responds to our demands for healthier, more natural foods, we will just have to avoid their over-processed products and the outlets that sell them.

Not buying the many unhealthful food choices available in supermarkets and restaurants will make you an advocate for a better food supply. Eating only Smart Foods will solve your weight issues while making a statement to the food industry that you are one of the many consumers demanding more healthy food options.

You might like the story below about an older woman who lost weight on the Smart for Life program. After a long lifetime of eating the Wrong Foods, she became inspired to avoid industrialized foods in favor of a healthy diet.

Jane E.

After her husband's death, Jane E. moved to a retirement community where she found companionship and comfort. However, her diet was suffering. She lived on convenience foods and packaged products she could heat up instantly in the microwave. With nobody to cook for, Jane did not want to take the time to cook for herself.

Jane knew that her food habits were unwise because she was gaining weight and had several ailments related to her overweight condition. Her energy was low, and she found herself huffing and puffing at the slightest exertion.

One night Jane attended a dinner party. An attractive and slender woman across the table mentioned that she had lost a lot of weight easily "by eating a little cookie." Jane was intrigued. The woman was 80 years old! Everyone knows how hard it is to lose weight at that age.

Jane asked her new friend for details, and that's how she learned about Smart for Life.

At the time, Jane was 77 years old herself. She weighed 196 pounds. "Very scary to me!" she admits now. "So close to 200!"

But until she heard about Smart for Life, Jane did not believe she could actually lose the weight she needed to lose. She knew that, as we age, the body's metabolism gradually declines. When we are in our 70s and 80s, if we are sedentary and not eating properly, it is next to impossible to achieve and maintain a healthy weight.

Jane realized that, if Smart for Life could help her older friend, it might just work for her. So she followed the program and destocked her kitchen, getting rid of shelf-stable foods and Wrong Foods made with artificial ingredients. She began to cook for herself: steaming vegetables, tossing fresh salads, and grilling lean fish or chicken. Sometimes she invited her new friend over for dinner, and the two women often shared Smart recipes.

In only four months, Jane lost 26 pounds. She improved her eating habits, her lifestyle, her body, and her health. "Goal!" says Jane E., living proof you can be Smart for Life at any age.

So there you have it: the Smart for Life story. You now hold in your hands the weight loss program that will work for you just like it did—and does to this day—for me and for thousands of my patients. You have in your hands all the benefits of our experience. Plus, you won't have to do all the research I had to do to find a safe and effective program that allows for permanent weight loss. You won't have to create your own weight loss products. I've done all that for you.

As you know, when I founded Smart for Life I based the diet and lifestyle program on my own years of struggle and, finally, success. Over the years since I established the first Smart for Life Weight Management Center, I have continued to develop new Smart food products for myself and my patients. In fact, I am always working on new ideas, creating different Smart foods and beverages that can aid in weight loss and help us keep the pounds off, and I am constantly updating my recipe files to include the most delicious and healthy Smart dishes. So you now can have access to anything new we come up with as well.

Since the first Smart for Life Weight Management Center opened its doors, I've worked with thousands of overweight people. My patients have lost as little as 10 pounds and as much as 200-plus pounds. My patients have told me what works and what doesn't, what tastes good and what they don't like. I am still listening and creating new products, new recipes and menus, to suit my patients' needs and desires. You may share in these ongoing developments. Visit my website and email me with ideas and input. I'd love to hear from you. (See the Appendix for my website landing page, locations, and contact information.)

When I lost weight quickly on what would become the Smart for Life program, I thought to myself, *Wow! Finally, a diet that tastes good and really works. Now I have a tool that will allow me to lose weight and maintain the right weight forever.*

Soon after I opened the first Smart for Life Weight Management Center in Boca Raton, Florida, the clinic was packed. My patients lost weight and discovered what I had found out: losing weight and keeping it off with Smart for Life was something they could do after all. My patients were extremely pleased. They told all their friends, and some of them signed up at Smart for Life, too. We had lines out the door as people waited to sign up for the program because the word was out: finally, a diet that tastes good, is healthy, and really works.

And now you know how to be Smart for Life, too.

Your Menu Plans

After I created the first Smart for Life cookie, I devised the weight loss program I planned to follow: six meals and snacks consisting of my special cookies plus a nice dinner with five servings of vegetables and 10 to 12 ounces of lean protein. The meals and snacks during the day were simple: I had my special cookies, and I carried them with me wherever I went. I also made sure to drink an 8-ounce glass of water with each meal and snack. I still drink water during the busy weekdays, and a cookie and water works great.

However, dinner was not so easy for me. I'm not the best cook, so I asked my wife Renata to help me with dinners. She is a wonderful and supportive person. Many of the ideas in this book came from her. But in this instance, she asked me to tell her *exactly what I would need.* She wanted a menu from me so she could be sure to serve just the right foods for the evening meals.

So Renata and I created a one week menu plan. She was able to utilize it to shop, cook, and plan out my dinners for a one week period. Then we repeated the one week cycle of menus, making changes where we wanted such as adding in more fresh fish and an occasional buffalo steak. We still use an updated version of that menu plan for our weekday dinner meals. My kids eat healthfully. My wife is trim and fit, too. We all benefit from eating Smart.

Now I will share with you an updated version of that one week menu plan. With input from nutritionists and my patients, I have created menus that should work for you. Feel free to individualize the following menus as you see fit. But please remember: Smart Foods only. Remember, you can replace any snack with a Smart For Life cookie or equivalent you baked yourself or bought. All dinners must have 2 to 5 serving of allowed vegetables we list it in the menu as a "salad," but you can be creative with vegetables as long as you follow our rules.

RCD Menu Plan

Day 1

BREAKFAST
2 hard-boiled egg whites with diced tomatoes and onions

SNACK
red and green bell pepper slices or Smart For Life cookie or equivalent

LUNCH
3 ounces steamed shrimp on 2 cups mixed greens

SNACK
Turkey Rollups: cucumber spears rolled into 2 1-ounce turkey slices or Smart For Life cookie or equivalent

DINNER
Tandoori Tofu* and Salad

SNACK
1/4 cup raw, unroasted, unsalted almonds or Smart For Life cookie or equivalent

Day 2

BREAKFAST
Scrambled Egg with Tofu*

SNACK
broccoli and cauliflower florets or Smart For Life cookie or equivalent

LUNCH
3 ounces grilled chicken breast with steamed vegetables

SNACK
1 ounce nonfat cheese or Smart For Life cookie or equivalent

DINNER
Fish Tacos* and salad

SNACK
raw baby carrots or Smart For Life cookie or equivalent

Day 3

BREAKFAST

2 scrambled egg whites

SNACK

1 cup shredded cabbage with balsamic vinegar or
Smart For Life cookie or equivalent

LUNCH

3 ounces canned tuna mixed with 1 tsp. fat-free mayo, tomato slices

SNACK

1/4 cup hummus with assorted raw veggies or Smart For Life cookie or equivalent

DINNER

"Fried" Quinoa (Smart Fried Rice)* and salad

SNACK

celery sticks and a Smart For Life Cookie

Day 4

BREAKFAST

1/4 cup fat-free plain Greek yogurt mixed with 1/4 cup blueberries, 1 tbsp. ground flaxseeds

SNACK

Dr. Sass's Kale Chips* or Smart For Life cookie or equivalent.

LUNCH

3 ounces broiled salmon on a bed of raw or cooked spinach

SNACK

2 hard-boiled egg whites or Smart For Life cookie or equivalent

DINNER

Blueberry Chicken* and salad

SNACK

raw bell pepper wedges or Smart For Life cookie or equivalent

Day 5

BREAKFAST

4 egg white omelet with steamed asparagus spears

SNACK

1/2 cup steamed edamame or Smart For Life cookie or equivalent

LUNCH

Greek Salad made with salad greens, 3 ounces grilled chicken strips, 1 ounce fat-free feta cheese, 3-5 black olives, balsamic vinegar

SNACK

1/4 cup raw, unroasted, unsalted cashews or Smart For Life cookie or equivalent

DINNER

Tuna Cucumber Boats* and salad

SNACK

1/4 cup fresh apple slices or Smart For Life cookie or equivalent

Day 6

BREAKFAST
Mini Mushroom Quiches* and salad

SNACK
steamed string beans or Smart For Life cookie or equivalent

LUNCH
3 ounces of grilled tofu with grilled eggplant slices or on top of salad greens

SNACK
1/2 cup fat-free plain Greek yogurt with 1/4 cup pomegranate slices or mixed berries or Smart For Life cookie or equivalent

DINNER
Grilled Rosemary-Salmon Skewers* and salad

SNACK
raw broccoli florets or Smart For Life cookie or equivalent

Day 7

BREAKFAST

2 ounces salmon salad made with 1 tsp. fat-free mayo, black pepper to taste

SNACK

chopped cucumbers and radishes or Smart For Life cookie or equivalent

LUNCH

Cobb Salad made with mixed salad greens,1 hard-boiled egg white, 2 ounces turkey breast

SNACK

2 ounces smoked salmon with sliced tomato or Smart For Life cookie or equivalent

DINNER

Steamed Clams or Mussels in Tomato Broth* and salad

SNACK

1 cup low-fat soy milk or Smart For Life cookie or equivalent

Once you reach your healthy weight goal, you might want to use the following one week menus to help you plan your meals and snacks. The new goal is to *eat Smart to maintain your goal weight.* This means continuing to practice the eating behaviors you have learned on the program: eating multiple small meals and snacks throughout the day, eating slowly and only when you are hungry, eating Smart Foods and avoiding the Wrong Foods.

My wife and I use a variation of the following Smart Maintenance menu plan for my evening meals during the week. On the weekends, we relax a little. Sometimes we dine out. But during the week, I eat mostly Smart for Life products during the day then a nice Smart dinner at night.

You can experiment with these menus to devise your own. See

what works for you, what makes you feel satisfied, what prevents you from feeling hungry. You will find yourself adding new recipes and new snack ideas to your menus over time. I still do. This keeps the menu evolving so that your meals are never boring.

Continue to weigh yourself once a week and record your weight in your Weight Chart. If you see that you have begun to gain weight, you'll need to make changes in your menu plan. I advise my patients who are on Smart Maintenance to keep recording in their Food Diary. You can use this tool and your Weight Chart (from the Appendix) to help you see what you may be doing wrong. Again, many of my patients continue using Smart For Life cookies or other products once or twice during the day to help control hunger and save calories.

Smart Maintenance Menu Plan

Day 1

BREAKFAST
Mini Mushroom Quiches*
(2 mini quiches equals 1 serving)

SNACK
1/4 cup hummus with assorted raw vegetables

LUNCH
4 ounce grilled chicken burger with large salad

SNACK
2 ounce fat-free cheese wedge

DINNER
Fish with Peppers, Tomatoes and Capers* and salad

SNACK
celery sticks with 1 tablespoon almond butter

Day 2

BREAKFAST

Mini Mushroom-Turkey Quiche*

SNACK

1/2 cup blueberries

LUNCH

4 ounce buffalo or soy burger topped with sautéed mushrooms and onions

SNACK

assorted raw vegetables

DINNER

Quinoa Jambalaya* and salad

SNACK

1/4 cup raw, unroasted, unsalted walnuts

Day 3

BREAKFAST
Pumpkin Frittata*

SNACK
raw spears of zucchini and yellow squash

LUNCH
Crab and Avocado Salad*

SNACK
1/2 cup fat-free Greek yogurt mixed with 2 tsp. old-fashioned oats
dash of cinnamon and nutmeg

DINNER
Stir Fry Chicken* and salad

SNACK
raw veggies and 3-5 black olives

Day 4

BREAKFAST

4 hard-boiled egg whites, 1/2 cup strawberries

SNACK

1/2 cup cherry tomatoes

LUNCH

Salmon Salad with Capers*

SNACK

2 ounces fat-free cheese

DINNER

Spaghetti and (Turkey) Meatballs* and salad

SNACK

dill pickle and a Smart For Life Cookie

Day 5

BREAKFAST
Muesli*

SNACK
Dr. Sass's Zucchini Chips*

LUNCH
Egg and Salmon Sandwich Wrap*

SNACK
2 ounces all-natural turkey breast with mustard

DINNER
Seared Tuna on Kale* and salad

SNACK
1/2 cup edamame

Day 6

BREAKFAST
Spinach-Tomato Omelet*

SNACK
seafood salad made with 2 ounces steamed shrimp, lobster or crab, fat-free mayo, diced celery and onion, sea salt and pepper to taste

LUNCH
Chopped Greek Salad with Chicken*

SNACK
1 ounce smoked salmon with sliced tomato and capers

DINNER
Calamari and Three Peppers* and salad

SNACK
1 cup almond milk

Day 7

BREAKFAST

Mini Vegetable Frittatas*

SNACK

cottage cheese-veggie salad with 2 ounces fat-free cottage cheese, diced radishes, celery, peppers, carrots, seasoned with ground pepper

LUNCH

Greek Tofu Salad*

SNACK

1/4 cup raw, unroasted, unsalted pumpkin seeds

DINNER

Chicken Marsala* and salad

SNACK

Homemade Frozen Fruit Popsicle*

If you have a food addiction or discover you are unable to resist the temptation to indulge in the Wrong Foods, you might benefit from the Fixed Meal Plan. I use this program with some of my patients who require a restrictive diet plan to kick-start their weight loss. Once their hunger is under control and some pounds have been shed, my patients find they can move on from the strict diet plan to the RCD. Usually a couple weeks on the Fixed Meal Plan will provide the limited focus and weight loss jump-start necessary for long-term success.

Here is the Fixed Meal Plan we use at the Smart for Life Weight Management Centers. *Do not deviate from this plan. Eat exactly what is included in the exact amounts given.*

Fixed Meal Plan

DAY 1-7: ***Every day you will choose from the following items for breakfast, lunch, and all snacks. Only your dinners will vary.***

BREAKFAST

Choose from one of following: Smart for Life cookie, muffin, shake, cereal, or other hunger-suppressing product

Midmorning SNACK

Choose from one of following: Smart for Life cookie, muffin, shake, cereal, soup, or other hunger-suppressing product

LUNCH

Choose from one of following: Smart for Life cookie, muffin, shake, cereal, soup, or other hunger-suppressing product

Midafternoon SNACK

Choose from one of following: Smart for Life cookie, muffin, shake, cereal, soup, or other hunger-suppressing product

Fixed Meal Plan

Late Afternoon SNACK

Choose from one of following: Smart for Life cookie, muffin, shake, cereal, soup, or other hunger-suppressing product

Bedtime Snack

Choose from one of following: Smart for Life cookie, muffin, shake, cereal, soup, or other hunger-suppressing product

DAY 1 DINNER

Fish with Peppers, Tomatoes and Capers* and salad

DAY 2 DINNER

Moroccan Turkey* and salad

DAY 3 DINNER

Sautéed Chicken Breast with Artichokes and Peppers* and salad

DAY 4 DINNER

Scallops with Capers and Tomatoes* and salad

DAY 5 DINNER

Chopped Greek Salad with Chicken* and salad

DAY 6 DINNER

Tilapia and Summer Vegetable Packets* and salad

DAY 7 DINNER

Crab Cakes* and salad

After two weeks successfully following the Fixed Meal Plan, you can think about whether you will now be able to control your eating behaviors so you can follow the RCD Menu Plan. If you do not feel you can take control of your eating, remain on the Fixed Meal Plan for another week or two and then reassess: has your hunger for Wrong Foods diminished? Are you obsessing less about the foods that put on weight and enjoying more the feeling of eating healthy? Are you losing weight? If so, you may be ready to switch to the RCD.

Try the RCD Menu Plan and see how you do. If you have trouble adhering to the RCD, you can return to the Fixed Meal Plan until you are psychologically and physically ready to take control of your eating behaviors—for life.

Smart for Life Recipes

The menu plans above include Smart Foods as main dishes, breakfast items, lunches, snacks, vegetable dishes, salads, beverages, and more. Here are all of the recipes you will need. Note that each of these recipes has been carefully coordinated with the RCD Menu Plan, the Smart Maintenance Menu Plan, and the Fixed Meal Plan. So if a dish is included on one of our Smart menu plans, the recipe has been included here.

The recipes that follow have been thoroughly tested and specially modified to make sure these choices are Smart and healthy as well as delicious. Plus, all of these Smart recipes are simple and affordable, saving you time in the kitchen and money in the supermarket.

If you don't already know this, you'll soon learn what I did: Smart Food is always easy, and fresh food always tastes best.

Breakfast Recipes:

Scrambled Egg with Tofu

(Makes 1 serving)

2 egg whites

1/2 tsp. dried tarragon

1/2 tsp. dried basil

dash of hot sauce

freshly ground pepper

1 tsp. olive oil

2 tbsp. crumbled tofu

Blend egg whites, tarragon, basil, hot sauce, and pepper in a small bowl. Mix with a fork. Add olive oil to skillet and heat over medium-low heat. Add tofu and cook, stirring, until warmed through (20-30 seconds). Add egg white mixture and stir until set but still creamy (20-30 seconds). Serve hot.

Calories: 140; Protein: 9 grams

Mini Mushroom Quiches

(Makes 12 servings)

2 tsp. olive oil

8 ounces low-fat soy meat alternative (sausage or burger)

8 ounces fresh mushrooms, sliced

1/4 cup sliced scallions

1/4 cup shredded fat-free cheese

1 tsp. freshly ground pepper

9-11 egg whites

1/4 cup water

Position rack in center of oven; preheat to 325 degrees. Grease muffin tin with a little bit of olive oil. Heat the rest of the olive oil in a large skillet over medium-high heat. Add soy meat and cook until golden brown (6-8 minutes). Transfer to a bowl to cool. Add mushrooms to skillet and cook, stirring often, until golden brown (5-7 minutes). Transfer mushrooms to the bowl with the soy meat. Let cool for 5 minutes. Stir in scallions, cheese, and pepper.

Whisk egg whites and water in a medium bowl. Divide the egg mixture evenly among the prepared muffin cups. Sprinkle a heaping tablespoon of the mushroom mixture into each cup.

Bake until the tops are just beginning to brown (25 minutes). Let cool on a wire rack for 5 minutes. Place a rack on top of the pan, flip it over, and turn the quiches out onto the rack. Turn upright and let cool completely.

Make Ahead Tip: Individually wrap mini quiches in plastic wrap and refrigerate for up to 3 days or freeze for up to 1 month. Reheat before serving.

Calories: 90; Protein: 9 grams

Mini Mushroom-Turkey Quiches*

(Makes 12 mini quiches; one per serving)

9 ounces ground white turkey (or chicken or soy meat)

2 tsp. extra-virgin olive oil

8 ounces fresh mushrooms, sliced

1/4 cup sliced scallions

1/4 cup shredded low-fat Swiss or mozzarella cheese

1 tsp. freshly ground pepper

10 egg whites

1 cup skim milk

Position rack in center of oven; preheat to 325 degrees. Grease a muffin tin with a little bit of olive oil. Heat a large skillet over medium-high heat. Add ground turkey or chicken or soy meat and cook until golden brown (6-8 minutes). Transfer to a bowl to cool. Add remaining olive oil to the pan. Add mushrooms and cook, stirring often, until golden brown (5-7 minutes). Transfer mushrooms to the bowl with the ground turkey. Let cool for 5 minutes. Stir in scallions, cheese, and pepper.

Whisk egg whites and milk in a medium bowl. Divide the egg mixture evenly among the prepared muffin cups. Sprinkle a heaping tablespoon of the turkey mixture into each cup.

Bake until the tops are just beginning to brown (25 minutes). Let cool on a wire rack for 5 minutes. Place a rack on top of the pan, flip it over and turn the quiches out onto the rack. Turn upright and let cool completely.

Calories: 80; Protein: 14 grams

Pumpkin Frittata*

(Makes 6 servings)

1 tbsp. olive oil

1 large carrot, shredded

1/4 cup thinly sliced scallions

2 garlic cloves, minced

10 egg whites

1/2 cup canned organic pumpkin puree or freshly cooked pumpkin

1/2 tsp. ground ginger

1/2 tsp. sea salt

1/4 tsp. pepper

1/8 tsp. nutmeg

1/2 cup shredded fat-free mozzarella

Preheat oven to 400 degrees. In a large skillet, warm 1 tsp. olive oil over medium heat. Add carrot, scallions, and garlic and cook, stirring frequently, until carrot is tender (about 5 minutes). Set aside to cool slightly.

In a medium bowl, stir together egg whites, pumpkin, ginger, salt, pepper and nutmeg. Blend, then stir into carrot mixture.

Warm the remaining 2 tsp. oil over medium heat in the skillet. Spoon in egg/carrot mixture and sprinkle with mozzarella cheese. Cook until bottom is set (about 5 minutes).

Transfer skillet to oven and bake until frittata is set (about 10 minutes). Serve in wedges direct from the skillet.

Calories: 150; Protein: 12 grams

Muesli*

(Makes 2 servings)

1/3 cup old-fashioned oats

1/2 cup nonfat plain Greek yogurt

1 tbsp. ground flax seeds

1 tbsp. crushed almonds

1 tsp. cinnamon

1/2 cup blueberries

Combine oats and yogurt. Mix in flax seeds, almonds and cinnamon. Toss in berries. Refrigerate overnight. Sweeten with stevia, if desired.

Calories: 130; Protein: 14 grams

Spinach-Tomato Omelet*

(Makes 4 servings)

2 tsp. extra-virgin olive oil

8 cherry tomatoes, halved

2 scallions, sliced

2 cups baby spinach, washed, with water still clinging to leaves

8 egg whites

1/4 cup shredded reduced-fat Cheddar cheese

pinch of sea salt

freshly ground pepper

1-2 tsp. water

Add oil to a skillet and heat over medium-high heat. Add tomatoes and scallions and cook, stirring once or twice, until softened (1-2 minutes). Place spinach on top, cover, and let wilt for 30 seconds. Stir to combine.

Add egg whites and reduce heat to medium-low and continue cooking, stirring constantly until the egg is starting to set (about 20 seconds). Continue cooking, lifting the edges so the uncooked egg will flow underneath, until mostly set (about 30 seconds more).

Sprinkle with cheese, salt, and pepper. Lift up an edge of the omelet and drizzle enough water under it so that the egg does not stick. Cover, reduce heat to low and cook until the egg is completely set and the cheese is melted (around 2 minutes). Fold over and serve.

Calories: 80; Protein: 9 grams

Mini Vegetable Frittatas*

(Makes 9 mini frittatas; 3 mini frittatas equals 1 serving)

10 egg whites

2 tbsp. fat-free milk or Zilch

1 ounce fat-free cheese, crumbled

1 cup diced tomato

2 cups chopped broccoli

sea salt and pepper

olive oil

Mix eggs and milk in a bowl. Add cheese and chopped vegetables. Season with salt and pepper. Spoon mixture into muffin tins coated with olive oil. Bake at 350 degrees for about 15 minutes or until set and golden on top.

Make Ahead Tip: you can refrigerate and reheat for a quick breakfast or snack.

Calories: 140; Protein: 14 grams

<u>Lunch Recipes:</u>

Crab and Avocado Salad*

(Makes 4 servings)

2/3 cup fat-free plain Greek yogurt

3 tbsp. fat-free mayo

1 tbsp. lemon juice

1/2 cup chopped chives

1/2 cup chopped fresh basil

fresh pepper and sea salt

1/2 pound crabmeat, diced

1 avocado, diced

3-4 cups romaine, chopped

1/2 pound string beans, steamed

1 cup cherry tomatoes

Puree yogurt, mayo, lemon juice, chives, and basil. Season with pepper and salt. In a bowl, mix crabmeat with half the avocado and 1 tbsp. of the yogurt mixture.

In a large bowl, combine romaine, remaining avocado, and string beans with the rest of the yogurt mixture. Divide into 4 portions on salad plates and top each with the crabmeat mixture. Decorate with tomatoes.

Calories: 314; Protein: 22 grams

Salmon Salad with Capers*

(Makes 2 servings)

7-1/2 ounce can salmon

2 tbsp. fat-free mayo

2 stalks celery, chopped

1 tbsp. capers

romaine lettuce

Combine salmon with mayo and celery. Stir in capers. Serve on a bed of lettuce.

Calories: 278; Protein 23 grams

Egg and Salmon Sandwich Wrap*

(Makes 1 serving: or 2 sandwich wraps)

2 tsp. extra-virgin olive oil

1 tbsp. finely chopped red onion

3 large egg whites, beaten

pinch of sea salt

1/2 teaspoon capers, rinsed and chopped (optional)

1 ounce smoked salmon

4 tomato slices

2 large lettuce leaves

Heat oil in a skillet over medium heat. Add onion and cook, stirring, until it begins to soften (less than 1 minute). Add egg whites, salt, and capers and cook, stirring constantly, until whites are set (about 30 seconds).

Layer the egg whites and smoked salmon between tomato slices and wrap in lettuce leaf.

Calories: 367; Protein: 32 grams

Chopped Greek Salad with Chicken*

(Makes 2 servings)

1/3 cup red wine vinegar

2 tbsp. extra-virgin olive oil

1 tbsp. chopped fresh dill (or 1 teaspoon dried oregano)

1 tsp. garlic powder

1/4 tsp. sea salt

1/4 tsp. freshly ground pepper

6 cups chopped romaine lettuce

2 1/2 cups chopped cooked chicken

2 tomatoes, chopped

1 cucumber, peeled, seeded and chopped

1/2 cup finely chopped red onion

1/2 cup sliced ripe black olives

1/2 cup crumbled fat-free feta cheese

Whisk vinegar, oil, dill (or oregano), garlic powder, salt, and pepper in a large bowl. Add remaining ingredients and toss until well coated.

Calories: 150; Protein: 15 grams

Greek Tofu Salad*

(Makes 2 servings)

1/3 cup crumbled feta cheese

1/4 cup chopped red onion or scallion

12 Kalamata (black) olives, pitted and chopped

3 tbsp. lemon juice

1 tbsp. extra-virgin olive oil

1 1/2 tsp. dried oregano

8 ounces firm tofu, drained and crumbled (1 cup)

sea salt and black pepper

1 ripe tomato, coarsely chopped

1 small cucumber, coarsely chopped

2 tbsp. chopped fresh parsley

In a medium bowl, combine feta, onion (or scallion), olives, lemon juice, oil, and oregano. Add tofu and mash together with a fork. Season with salt and pepper. Cover and refrigerate for 20 minutes.

Add tomato, cucumber and parsley. Add more salt and pepper if needed.

Calories: 300; Protein: 20 grams

Dinner Recipes:

Tandoori Tofu*

(Makes 3 servings)

2 tsp. paprika

1 tsp. salt

1/2 tsp. ground cumin

1/2 tsp. ground coriander

1/4 tsp. ground turmeric

3 tbsp. extra-virgin olive oil

1 tbsp. minced garlic

1 tbsp. lime juice

2 14-ounce packages extra-firm or firm tofu, drained

2/3 cup nonfat plain Greek yogurt

6 tbsp. sliced scallions or chopped fresh cilantro for garnish

Preheat grill to medium-high. Combine paprika, 1/2 teaspoon salt, cumin, coriander, and turmeric in a small bowl. Heat oil in a small skillet over medium heat. Add garlic, lime juice, and the spice mixture. Cook, stirring, until sizzling and fragrant (about 1 minute). Remove from the heat.

Slice each tofu block crosswise into 6 slices; pat dry. Use about 3 tablespoons of the hot, spiced oil to brush both sides of the tofu slices; sprinkle with the remaining 1/2 teaspoon salt. Reserve the remaining spiced oil.

Oil the grill rack (see Tip below). Grill the tofu until it has grill marks and is heated through (typically 2 to 3 minutes per side).

In a small serving bowl, combine yogurt with the reserved spiced oil. Serve the grilled tofu topped with the yogurt sauce and garnish with scallions (or cilantro) if desired.

Calories: 346; Protein: 24 grams

Fish Tacos*

(Makes 4 servings)

1 tbsp. olive oil

1 lb. tilapia fillets

sea salt and pepper

1/2 cup fat-free plain Greek yogurt

2 tbsp. lime juice

1 clove garlic, minced

4 large lettuce leaves

1 cup shredded cabbage

1/4 cup salsa

Heat oil in a medium sized skillet. Add fish and season with salt and pepper. Stir-fry over medium-high heat until thoroughly cooked.

Combine yogurt, lime juice and garlic. Place each fish fillet on a lettuce leaf and top with a scoop of cabbage. Drizzle with yogurt mixture. Serve hot with salsa. Calories: 270; Protein: 29 grams

“Fried” Quinoa (Smart Fried Rice)*

(Makes 1 serving)

1/2 cup water

1 cup quinoa, cooked according to package instructions (use 1/2 cup cooked for recipe and store rest in refrigerator)

1/4 onion, chopped

1 carrot, diced

1 stalk celery, diced

1 clove garlic, minced

1/4 red bell pepper

1 tsp. low-sodium soy sauce

3 large egg whites

1/2 cup broccoli, chopped

Heat 2 tbsp. water in a medium sized skillet. Add onions and carrots and steam for a few minutes. Add remaining ingredients except for broccoli. Cover and cook for about 3 minutes.

Add the 1/2 cup cooked quinoa; add broccoli and the remaining water to the skillet. Cover and steam for several minutes or until broccoli turns bright green.

Variation: Add in other vegetables such as mushrooms, bamboo shoots, water chestnuts, and yellow squash; add cubed chicken, turkey, or shrimp.

Calories: 350; Protein: 25 grams

Renata's Blueberry Chicken*

(Makes 4 servings)

2 cups blueberries

1/2 cup pomegranate or blueberry juice

1/2 cup mustard

2 tbsp. olive oil

pinch of stevia

3 tbsp. dried rosemary

2 tbsp. dried basil

1 tbsp. black pepper

4-6 ounce skinless boneless chicken breasts

sea salt

pinch of garlic powder

In a blender, combine 1 cup berries, juice, mustard, olive oil, stevia, rosemary, basil, and pepper to make a marinade.

Season chicken with salt and garlic powder. Pour marinade over chicken and marinate in refrigerator for 4 hours or overnight.

Heat a large skillet and brown chicken. Add marinade and bring to a boil. Reduce heat and simmer about 20 minutes or until chicken is cooked.

Add remaining berries and serve hot.

Calories: 334; Protein: 34 grams

Tuna Cucumber Boats*

(Makes 1 serving)

olive oil

1 large cucumber

6-ounce can tuna

1 egg white

1/3 cup shredded carrot

1/4 cup grated onion

1/3 cup diced tomato, diced

1/3 cup leek, chopped

sea salt and pepper

Preheat oven to 350 degrees. Oil a baking sheet. Cut cucumber in half lengthwise. Combine tuna, egg white, carrots, onion, tomato, leeks, salt and pepper. Make 2 long patties the size of the cucumber halves. Place on baking sheet and bake for 20 minutes.

Use spatula to move fish patties onto the cucumber halves.

Variation: Substitute zucchini or tomato slices for the cucumber and make fish patties to fit

Calories: 200; Protein: 28 grams

Grilled Rosemary-Salmon Skewers*

(Makes 4 servings)

2 tsp. minced fresh rosemary

2 tsp. extra-virgin olive oil

2 cloves garlic, minced

1 tsp. freshly grated lemon zest

1 tsp. lemon juice

1/2 tsp. kosher salt

1/4 tsp. freshly ground pepper

1 lb. salmon, cut into 1-inch cubes

1 pint cherry tomatoes

Preheat grill to medium-high. Combine rosemary, oil, garlic, lemon zest, lemon juice, salt, and pepper in a medium bowl. Add salmon cubes and toss to coat. Alternate the salmon cubes and cherry tomatoes on eight 12-inch skewers.

Oil the grill rack and grill the skewers, carefully turning once. Cook until the salmon is cooked through (4-6 minutes total). Serve immediately.

Calories: 246; Protein: 23 grams

Steamed Clams or Mussels in Tomato Broth*

(Makes 1 serving)

1 14-1/2 ounce can diced tomatoes

1/2 cup water

1/2 cup chopped onion

1 tsp. minced garlic

2 tsp. dried basil

3 dozen clams or mussels, cleaned and scrubbed

fresh parsley, scallions or cilantro, chopped

Combine tomatoes, water, onion, garlic, and basil in a large pan. Bring to a boil. Add clams or mussels. Cover pan and cook until shells open.

Spoon into bowl and top with parsley, scallions or cilantro.

Calories: 300; Protein: 28 grams

Quinoa Jambalaya*

(Makes 1 serving)

1 tbsp. canola oil

1 onion, chopped

1 zucchini, chopped

1 red bell pepper, diced

1 tbsp. fresh garlic, minced

6 ounce skinless boneless chicken breast, diced

1/4 cup quinoa

1/2 cup organic chicken broth

1 can diced tomatoes

1/4 pound raw shrimp

2 stalks scallion, chopped

sea salt and pepper

Heat oil in large skillet over medium high heat. Add onion, zucchini, red pepper, and garlic. Heat for 2 minutes.

Add chicken and continue cooking for 5 minutes. Add quinoa, broth, and tomatoes. Bring to boil; reduce heat to simmer, cover skillet, and cook for 10 minutes.

Add shrimp and cook, covered, for another 3 minutes until shrimp is done but not overdone. Top with scallions and season to taste.

Calories: 400; Protein: 24 grams

Stir Fry Chicken*

(Makes 4 servings)

2 tsp. canola oil

1 tbsp. minced fresh ginger

2 tsp. fresh lemongrass, minced and peeled

2 cloves garlic, minced

1 lb. skinless boneless chicken breast, cut into bite-sized pieces

2 cups shelled edamame

2 cups assorted blanched vegetables (broccoli, cauliflower, bell peppers, bamboo shoots, onion, etc.)

2 tbsp. low-sodium soy sauce

1 tbsp. mirin (sweet rice wine)

1 tsp. dark sesame oil

1/2 cup scallions, chopped

2 tsp. dark sesame seeds

sea salt

Heat oil in a large skillet over medium-high heat. Add ginger, lemongrass, and garlic; sauté until soft (1-2 minutes). Add chicken, edamame, and vegetables; sauté for 3 minutes.

Combine soy sauce, mirin, and sesame oil. Add to skillet and cook for 1 minute. Remove from heat. Stir in scallions, sesame seeds, and salt to taste.

Serving Suggestion: Serve over quinoa or gluten-free mung bean pasta.

Calories: 400; Protein: 32 grams

Spaghetti and (Turkey) Meatballs*

(Makes 8 servings)

olive oil

1 onion, chopped

1/2 red pepper, chopped

1/2 green pepper, chopped

1 garlic clove, chopped

2 lbs. ground white-meat turkey

3 egg whites

1 tbsp. whole wheat bread crumbs

1 tsp. sea salt

1/4 tsp. black pepper

2 cups organic tomato sauce

2 pkgs. gluten-free black bean pasta, cooked according to package directions

Heat oil in large skillet. Add onion and stir-fry until onion yellows. Add peppers and cook until soft. Add garlic and stir-fry until brown. Remove from stove to cool for 10 minutes.

In a large bowl, mix together turkey, egg whites, bread crumbs, salt, and pepper. Add in stir-fried veggies and mix well.

Form 16 little meatballs by hand. Brown in the skillet over medium-high heat until cooked through.

Heat tomato sauce and pour over cooked pasta. Add meatballs and serve.

Calories: 410; Protein 44 grams

Seared Tuna on Kale*

(Makes 2 servings)

1 tbsp. orange juice

sea salt and pepper

2 cups kale, chopped

1/3 cup pomegranate seeds

2 4-ounce tuna steaks

2 tbsp. canola oil

In a medium bowl, toss together orange juice, salt, pepper, kale, and pomegranate seeds. Set salad aside.

Season tuna with salt and pepper. Heat canola oil in a large skillet. Add tuna and sear on both sides over high heat.

Place steaks on top of kale salad and serve.

Calories: 442; Protein 31 grams

Calamari and Three Peppers*

(Makes 4 servings)

2 lbs. calamari rings

1/2 red bell pepper, chopped

1/2 yellow bell pepper, chopped

1/2 orange bell pepper, chopped

1 tbsp. garlic, minced

1-2 fresh red chilies, minced

1 small onion, chopped

2 tbsp. ground coriander

2 tbsp. ground cumin

1 tbsp. fresh ginger

1 tbsp. chopped lemongrass

1 tsp. olive oil

1/4 cup chopped fresh cilantro

Combine calamari with peppers, garlic, chilies, and onion; set aside.

In a small mixing bowl, combine coriander, cumin, ginger, and lemongrass. Add to calamari mixture.

Heat oil in a skillet. Add calamari and vegetable mixture and stir-fry over medium heat for 15 minutes.

Garnish with cilantro and serve hot.

Calories: 264; Protein: 38 grams

Chicken Marsala*

(Makes 4 servings)

1 cup plain nonfat Greek yogurt

1/4 cup coarsely chopped fresh cilantro

3 tbsp. extra-virgin olive oil

1 tbsp. garam masala

2 tsp. sea salt

1 large garlic clove, pressed

4 6-ounce skinless boneless chicken breasts

2 small onions, cut into 1/4-inch thick slices

Mix yogurt, cilantro, olive oil, garam masala, salt, and garlic. Spread in a 13x9x2-inch glass baking dish.

Add chicken, 1 piece at a time, coating all sides with marinade. Cover with plastic wrap; refrigerate for at least 2 hours.

Preheat oven to 400 degrees. Arrange onions in a thin layer on a large rimmed baking sheet. Add chicken, arranged in single layer. Discard remaining marinade. Cook for 20-30 minutes. Serve on top of the onion slices; spoon pan juices over chicken. Calories: 395; Protein: 38 grams

Fish with Peppers, Tomatoes and Capers*

(Makes 4 servings)

2 tbsp. olive oil

4- 6 ounce fish fillets (tilapia, snapper, flounder, sole or mahi mahi)

sea salt and pepper

1 onion, chopped

1 red bell pepper, chopped

2 tomatoes, diced

2-3 tbsp. capers

1 tbsp. fresh garlic, minced

Heat oil in medium skillet over medium-high heat; season fish with salt and pepper. Heat fish until cooked throughout. Remove from skillet and set aside. Add onion and bell pepper to skillet; cook until soft. Add tomatoes, capers, and garlic; cook until soft.

Spoon vegetables onto fish fillets and serve.

Calories: 255; Protein: 35 grams

Moroccan Turkey*

(Makes 2 servings)

2 tbsp. olive oil

1 onion, chopped

1 clove garlic, minced

1/4 cup water

1/2-inch fresh ginger root, minced

6 whole cloves

1 tsp. ground cinnamon

1/2 tsp. star anise

1 tsp. fennel seeds

2 6-ounce boneless skinless turkey breasts, diced

1/2 cup shiitake mushrooms, chopped

6 stalks asparagus, chopped

Heat oil in large skillet over medium-high heat. Sauté onion and garlic until lightly browned. Add water, ginger, cloves, cinnamon, star anise, and fennel seeds. Reduce heat and simmer for 10 minutes.

Add turkey; cover skillet and simmer for 10 more minutes.

Stir in mushrooms and asparagus. Cover skillet and simmer until asparagus turns bright green.

Serving Suggestion: Delicious served over cooked quinoa.

Calories: 358; Protein 30 grams

Sautéed Chicken Breast with Artichokes and Peppers*

(Makes 4 servings)

4 tsp. extra-virgin olive oil

4 6-ounce boneless skinless chicken breasts

sea salt

freshly ground black pepper

1 onion, halved and sliced

4 cloves garlic, smashed

2 sprigs fresh thyme, leaves stripped

1-1/2 cups marinated artichokes, drained and patted dry

1/2 cup roasted red peppers, sliced into strips

1 cup organic chicken broth

1/4 cup flat leaf parsley leaves

Preheat the oven to 400 degrees. Heat olive oil in a large skillet over medium-high heat. Season the chicken with salt and pepper and brown until golden (about 4 minutes per side). Transfer the chicken to a roasting pan and bake until firm to the touch (about 10 minutes).

While chicken is baking, add onion, garlic, and thyme to the skillet and cook, stirring occasionally, until brown (about 5 minutes). Add artichokes and roasted peppers; cook until brown (about 3 minutes). Add the broth and bring to a full boil. Turn down to simmer and add parsley. Add salt and pepper to taste.

Pour the sauce over the chicken, and serve.

Calories: 515; Protein: 44 grams

Scallops with Capers and Tomatoes*

(Makes 4 servings)

12 large sea scallops,

1 tbsp. olive oil

1 clove garlic, minced

1/4 cup tomato puree

1/4 cup water

1 tomato, diced

3 tbsp. capers

2 tbsp. fresh basil, chopped

sea salt

black pepper

Rinse and dry scallops. Add oil to a large skillet and heat over medium-high heat. Add scallops and cook for 3 minutes on each side. Remove from skillet and set aside.

Add remaining ingredients to the skillet. Simmer until heated. Spoon broth over scallops and serve.

Calories: 212; Protein: 29 grams

Chopped Greek Salad with Chicken*

(Makes 1 serving)

1/3 cup red-wine vinegar

2 tbsp. extra-virgin olive oil

1 tbsp. chopped fresh dill (or 1 tsp. dried oregano)

1 tsp. garlic powder

1/4 tsp. sea salt

1/4 tsp. freshly ground pepper

6 cups chopped romaine lettuce

2-1/2 cups chopped cooked chicken

2 tomatoes, chopped

1 cucumber, peeled, seeded and chopped

1/2 cup finely chopped red onion

1/2 cup sliced black olives

1/2 cup crumbled fat-free feta cheese

Whisk together vinegar, oil, dill (or oregano), garlic powder, salt, and pepper in a large bowl. Add rest of ingredients and toss to coat.

Calories: 343; Protein: 31 grams

Tilapia and Summer Vegetable Packets*

(Makes 4 servings)

1 cup quartered cherry tomatoes

1 cup diced summer squash

1 cup thinly sliced red onion

12 green beans, cut into 1-inch pieces

1/4 cup pitted and coarsely chopped black olives

2 tbsp. lemon juice

1 tbsp. chopped fresh oregano

1 tbsp. extra-virgin olive oil

1 tsp. capers, rinsed

1/4 tsp. sea salt

1/4 tsp. freshly ground pepper

4 6-ounce tilapia fillets

sea salt and pepper

Preheat grill to medium. Combine all ingredients except fish in a large bowl.

Put 2 20-inch sheets of foil on top of one another (a double layer will help prevent burning) and drizzle with olive oil. Place one fillet in the center of the foil. Sprinkle with salt and pepper then top with about 3/4 cup of the vegetable mixture. Bring the short ends of the foil together, leaving enough room in the packet for steam to gather and cook the food. Fold the foil over and pinch to seal. Pinch seams together along the sides. Make sure all the seams are tightly sealed to keep steam from escaping.

Repeat with more foil and the remaining fillets; season and add the vegetable mixture to each before folding into foil packets.

Grill the packets for 5-6 minutes or until the fish is cooked through and the vegetables are just tender.

Carefully open both ends of the packets to allow steam to escape. Use a spatula to slide the contents onto plates and serve hot.

Variation: Instead of grilling, preheat oven to 425 degrees. Bake the packets directly on an oven rack for 20-25 minutes or until the tilapia is cooked through and the vegetables are just tender.

Calories: 181; Protein: 24 grams

Crab Cakes*

(Makes 3 servings)

1 lb. crab, cut in small pieces

2 egg whites, lightly beaten

2 tbsp. organic panko (Japanese-style bread crumbs) or Smart for Life bagel chips

1/4 cup fat-free mayonnaise

2 tbsp. minced chives

2 stalks celery, diced

1 tbsp. Dijon mustard

1 tbsp. lemon juice

1 tsp. celery seed

1 tsp. onion powder

1/4 tsp. freshly ground pepper

3-4 dashes hot sauce

1 tbsp. extra-virgin olive oil

In a large bowl, mix crab with rest of ingredients except for olive oil. Form by hand into 3 large patties or 6 smaller patties.

Heat oil in a large skillet over medium heat. Cook the patties until golden brown.

Serve on a bed of greens such as fresh arugula or spinach.

Calories 326; Protein: 32 grams

Snack Recipes:

Dr. Sass's Kale Chips*

1 head of fresh kale

2 tbsp. olive oil

sea salt and pepper

Preheat an oven to 350 degrees. Line a cookie sheet with parchment paper or aluminum foil. Coat with 1 tsp. of the olive oil.

With a knife or kitchen shears, carefully remove kale leaves from the thick stems; tear leaves into bite-size pieces. Wash and thoroughly dry (you can use a salad spinner). Drizzle with remaining olive oil and sprinkle with salt and pepper.

Bake for 10-15 minutes or until the edges are browned but not burned.

Cool before eating.

Depending on the size of the head of kale, this recipe makes a lot of chips. Save extras in a Ziploc plastic bag.

Homemade Frozen Fruit Popsicles*

fresh fruit

water

Puree fruit in blender. (Pomegranate, berries, grapes, pineapple, or other fruits may be blended together). Add enough water to achieve desired consistency.

Pour into ice trays and freeze.

For a refreshing snack, remove from ice tray and eat like a popsicle.

Dr. Sass's Flaxseed Crackers

(Makes 12)

olive oil

1 cup flax meal

1/2 tsp. sea salt

1/4 tsp. black pepper

water

2 tbsp. sesame seeds

Preheat oven to 350 degrees. Spread parchment paper on a baking sheet and grease lightly with olive oil.

Place flax meal in a large mixing bowl and add salt and pepper. Add in water slowly, stirring, until the consistency of thick pancake batter.

Spread thin on parchment paper. Sprinkle with sesame seeds.

Bake for 5-10 minutes or until crisp. Cool and cut into squares.

Dr. Sass's Zucchini Chips

(Makes 4 servings)

3 tbsp. olive oil

2 medium zucchini, peeled and cut into 1/4-inch rounds

1 tbsp. oregano

2 tbsp. low-fat cheese

sea salt

black pepper

Preheat oven to 350 degrees. Lightly grease a baking sheet with a small amount of the olive oil.

In a large bowl, toss zucchini rounds with remaining olive oil. Add oregano and toss to coat.

Arrange zucchini in a single layer on the baking sheet. Sprinkle with cheese.

Bake for 30-40 minutes or until golden brown.

Season with salt and pepper and serve warm or cool.

Dressing Recipes:

Renata's Balsamic Dressing

(Makes 1 serving)

1/2 cup balsamic vinegar

2 tbsp. Dijon mustard

1 clove garlic, minced

sea salt

black pepper

In a medium-sized bowl, combine vinegar with mustard and garlic. Add salt and pepper to taste. Mix until well blended.

Variation: For thicker dressing, add additional mustard.

Smart Salad Dressing

(Makes 1 serving)

2 tbsp. red wine vinegar

1/4 tsp. dried oregano

1/4 tsp. sea salt

1/4 tsp. black pepper

In a mixing bowl, whisk all ingredients together until well blended.

<u>Vegetable Dish Recipes:</u>

Asparagus Pepper Salad

(Makes 2 servings)

1 cup asparagus, cut into 1-inch pieces

1/2 cup green bell pepper, chopped

1/2 cup red bell pepper, chopped

1/2 cup yellow bell pepper, chopped

2 green onions, thinly sliced

1/3 cup Renata's Balsamic Dressing or commercial, all-natural vinaigrette

In a medium-size saucepan, boil asparagus for 3 minutes. Drain and cool.

In a medium bowl, mix peppers, onion, and dressing. Stir in asparagus and mix to coat.

Refrigerate for 3-4 hours before serving.

Sautéed Kale

(Makes 4 servings)

2 heads kale

3 tbsp. canola oil

4 cloves garlic, finely chopped

1/2 tsp. sea salt

1/2 tsp. black pepper

1 tbsp. fresh lemon juice

Rinse kale; pat dry. (You can use a salad spinner, if desired). Remove stems and cut leaves into 1/4-inch strips.

Heat oil in a large skillet. Add garlic and cook over medium-high heat, stirring, for 30 seconds.

Add half the chopped greens and cook, stirring, until they begin to wilt. Add remainder of greens and cook, stirring, for 10 minutes or until tender.

Remove from heat and season with salt, pepper, and lemon juice. Serve hot.

Mango Chutney

(Makes 1-2 cups)

5 dried serrano chilies

1 large ripe mango

3 dried apricots

2 tbsp. lime juice

2 tsp. ground cayenne pepper

2 tsp. ground coriander

1 tsp. ground cumin

1 tsp. ground ginger

1/4 tsp. ground cloves

1/4 tsp. ground nutmeg

Remove seeds and stems from chilies; chop into tiny pieces.

Peel and chop mango.

Soak apricots in warm water to soften; chop into tiny pieces.

Put all ingredients in a blender and puree.

Allow to sit for 6-12 hours before serving.

Serving Suggestion: Use sparingly as a dip or dressing with fish, chicken, and vegetable dishes.

Cauliflower Mash

(Makes 2 servings)

1/2 small head cauliflower

2 cups organic chicken or vegetable broth

1 tbsp. minced garlic

1/2 tsp. sea salt

1/4 tsp. black pepper

Break cauliflower into bite-size florets.

In a large saucepan, bring broth to a boil. Add garlic and florets and simmer until cauliflower is fork-tender.

Place cauliflower in a bowl; set broth aside. Season vegetables with salt and pepper. Whip or mash, adding broth gradually, to achieve mashed potato consistency.

Serve hot.

Beverage Recipes:

Healthy Smoothies

(Makes 2 servings)

1 ripe banana

1/2 cup plain low-fat yogurt

1/2 cup fruit (e.g., berries, sliced apple, mango chunks, sliced peaches)

4 ice cubes, optional

Blend all ingredients in blender until smooth. Use ice for a slushy drink.

Antioxidant Smoothie

(Makes 2 servings)

1 ripe banana

1/2 cup plain low-fat yogurt

1/2 cup grapes

1/2 cup blueberries

4 ice cubes

Blend all ingredients in blender until smooth.

Banana Coffee Smoothie

(Makes 2 servings)

2 small ripe bananas

1 cup low-fat almond milk

1 cup plain nonfat yogurt

1/4 cup strong coffee

1/4 tsp. ground cinnamon

dash nutmeg

Blend all ingredients in blender until smooth.

Flaxseed and Fruit Smoothie

(Makes 2 servings)

1 ripe banana

3 cups low-fat soy milk

1 tbsp. ground flaxseed

1/4 tsp. ground cinnamon

dash nutmeg

1/4 cup berries or chopped fruit (e.g., mango, guava, papaya, pomegranate)

Blend all ingredients in blender until smooth.

Cooking Tips

How you prepare your food is important. You may need to make some significant changes in your cooking techniques. My wife is Polish, and she often roasted large cuts of meat. That is the way her family eats, and her culture is centered around this kind of food. However, eating red meat is not healthy and puts the weight on me. So my wife cooks in a manner that is more healthful for the whole family. Only on special occasions do we have a big Polish feast.

The key to healthy cooking is to reduce or eliminate sugar and other high glycemic index ingredients, limit unhealthy fats and calories while adding nutrition without sacrificing taste and flavor. Read over any new recipes carefully and think about how you might improve them. You may have to experiment until you find recipes you like that are Smart.

Here are the cooking tips I share with my patients at the Smart for Life Weight Management Centers:

Tip #1: Get a blender or food processor to help make smoothies, soups, and other Smart Foods.

Tip #2: Get a salad spinner to clean your fresh greens. It's fast and easy.

Tip #3: Buy packaged prewashed greens for quickie salads. Wash once more in the salad spinner.

Tip #4: Shave your veggies into the thinnest slices to make portions seem larger.

Tip #5: Substitute vegetable or chicken broth for butter and sauté in wine or broth.

Tip #6: Marinate in wine, broth, or homemade dressing with herbs.

Tip #7: All the foods you like fried can be baked or grilled instead—toss your food into a clean ziplock bag with a beaten egg white then roll in finely ground flaxseed cracker crumbs, arrange on a baking sheet, and bake until done.

Tip #8: Use 2 egg whites instead of 1 whole egg in all recipes.

Tip #9: Give your egg yolks to your plants; dilute in water and feed to the indoor or outdoor shrubs, trees, or other greenery and watch how they grow.

Tip #10: In recipes, use skim milk instead of whole, 2% or 1% fat; you won't notice the difference.

Tip #11: Use fat-free sour cream instead of regular sour cream in recipes and as a dip for vegetables.

Tip #12: Use a vegetable oil sprayer to reduce the amount of oil you use in cooking; cooking sprays are full of nasty additives, so avoid them.

Tip #13: Make your own salad dressing with olive oil, balsamic vinegar, fresh herbs, and spices.

Tip #14: Explore new vegetables, different kinds of fish and seafood, unusual cuts of chicken. Try some almond milk, soy milk, or low-fat yogurt. Be daring and creative.

Bon appétit!

Before we move on to the fact-packed science sections of *Smart for Life: Dr. Sass's Solution*, you might want to read the following story about a health professional like myself who used Smart for Life to solve some serious personal and professional issues around weight.

Anne-Marie C.

Since Anne-Marie C. works as a dietitian in a medical center, she knows a lot about nutrition. Healthy food and balanced diets make up the foundation of her profession. She is a knowledgeable and skilled professional.

However, in 2006 Anne-Marie suffered a miscarriage. She became depressed and allowed herself to indulge her ravenous sweet tooth. She did not follow her own nutrition standards and ate for emotional reasons. The weight piled on. Over the next few years, Anne-Marie gained between 50 and 60 pounds.

In December of 2008, Anne-Marie went on a vacation with her family to Disney World where she watched her obese mother struggle to walk around the theme park. "I got scared," Anne-Marie admits. She was aware that her own blood pressure was elevated. Not good for someone in her 20s.

After looking at photos from the vacation, "I became disgusted with myself," Anne-Marie says. "I knew what I had to do."

A co-worker suggested the Smart for Life program. Nutritionists know a healthy diet is the only way to lose excess body fat and preserve lean muscle tissue. Nutrition professionals are well aware that fad diets are unhealthy and unsuccessful in the long run because our bodies need proper nutrition and adequate energy to function properly. When Anne-Marie C. researched Smart for Life, she liked what she saw: a healthy, organic diet plan that allowed for permanent weight loss while changing undesirable eating behaviors.

As a nutrition professional, Anne-Marie chose to monitor herself on the diet program. She ordered Smart for Life products online and adhered to the program. Right away she found that the weight loss plan "helped to curb my sweet tooth and stopped me from wanting to snack by allowing me to eat every 3 to 4 hours." She was attentive to portion size, and she chose her foods carefully.

Anne-Marie's weight dropped steadily over the course of 15 months. She lost 66 pounds and now fits into a size 8 dress. Her blood pressure has returned to normal, and her BMI has dropped from 37 to 25. "Smart for Life gave me more energy, self-confidence, and love for myself again."

She started playing tennis, a sport she had dropped after her weight gain. She was able to balance her diet and exercise, eating in moderation and gradually improving her fitness level. She noticed that her metabolism had changed and was more efficient. "I stayed full longer, which improved my tennis game," she says.

Anne-Marie continues to lose weight on the Smart for Life program. "I think I have finally managed to find a good balance with eating, exercise, and Smart for Life products. I indulge (in moderation) when I want to, but most of the time I follow the Smart for Life program."

Anne-Marie's weight goal includes fitting into a size 6. Recently, she added a running program to her activities. "I never had the endurance for running before," she says. With the weight loss, things have changed: she ran her first 5K and loved the experience.

Understandably, Anne-Marie C. is pleased with her success. She feels like she looks more professional because she practices what she preaches, and her personal life has benefitted as well. "My clothes are looser, I look sexier, and feel great. My husband hasn't seen me this happy in a long time. I feel beautiful again."

Part III: The Science of Being Smart for Life

"No disease that can be treated by diet should be treated with any other means."

—Maimonides

"We never repent of having eaten too little."

—Thomas Jefferson

Chapter 7: Get Smart

If you are on the Smart for Life program, as you certainly should be by now, you are not bored with the food you are eating. Am I right? I mean, I've been on the program for many years, and I'm not in the least bit bored. Day after day, I still find myself enjoying Smart Foods.

However, I am continuously improving my diet as I learn more about the influence of diet on health and disease. I'm constantly looking for new ways to incorporate Superfoods into my daily diet. I'm always combing the medical literature in search of new Superfoods. When new research comes out in the medical literature, I want to know about it.

Smart for Life is always improving and expanding. I continue to develop healthy new products that taste great and support safe weight loss. I'm diligently reading the latest research in the field of nutrition to discover functional ingredients I might add to my own diet—and to Smart for Life food products—ingredients that will benefit me—and you. I'm on the lookout for studies on foodstuffs that may contribute to improved cardiac function, stable blood sugar and insulin levels, better digestive function, boosts in immunity and longevity. When the evidence is in, I begin to devise ways of adding effective functional ingredients to my diet and then to our line of Smart Food products.

Since I lost weight with my first Smart for Life cookie made with organic ingredients, I have continued to develop an ever-expanding line of healthy weight loss products to provide dieters with both variety and convenience. There are Smart for Life muffins and protein bars as well as soups, cereals, beverages, and more. There are fun food products for kids and nutritious, organic items that are Smart for any time in your life.

In fact, I'm working on some delicious new products right now that may be available by the time you read this chapter. The science of nutrition is continually revealing new links between our diets and our health. I am learning as I go, and I am sharing what I find out with you.

One thing that will never change: I don't like to feel hungry. I know what that can lead to: cranky mood, lack of energy, and over-eating the Wrong Foods. So I make sure to follow the Smart for Life program so I won't be hungry. You won't be hungry either because the Smart for Life program is designed to ensure you eat the right foods often enough to keep your appetite in check.

To assist with the hunger problem that so commonly defeats dieters, however, I have added functional ingredients to Smart for Life products, special ingredients that provide a feeling of fullness and satiety and help to improve health. If your six small meals and snacks plus a healthy dinner are not quite filling enough, you might want to try Smart for Life cookies with LeptiCore or some of our special beverages. Take a look at our website and scan the product information to find items that will help you on your journey.

You should never be hungry on Smart for Life. This is key.

Perhaps the best thing about being on the Smart for Life program, however, is this: *your overall health will improve.* Being on the Smart for Life program will help to lower elevated blood sugar and cholesterol while improving digestion and gastrointestinal function. You won't be eating too much sugar, red meat, or over-processed foods. You won't be eating a lot of junk. Instead, you'll be eating a lot of nutrient-rich greens, veggies, and lean protein. If you are using

Smart for Life products, you will be including in your dietary intake some cutting-edge functional ingredients like plant sterols, omega-3 fatty acids, and super-fibers.

This means you will be eating the kind of foods that can improve your health and help you to live longer. The Smart for Life program not only results in safe and healthy weight loss, but being Smart will reduce your chances for developing chronic diseases and may slow the aging process.

And you won't blow through your food budget with Smart for Life. You should actually find you are spending less money on food because you no longer waste your hard-earned dollars on junk food, fast food, and over-processed, overpriced snacks. Plus, as your health improves, you will be spending less money on medical care. This is where the significant savings show up: reduced expenditures on prescription medications, doctor visits, over-the-counter remedies for this and that.

Be Smart, get fit, spend less on health care. Now, there's a solution the whole country could get behind.

If my experience is any guide, and I hope that it is, there is hope for you if you are overweight or obese. *You can lose weight and get healthy. There is a way.* If you follow my program, you will see results very quickly. And, like me, you will be hooked. You won't feel bored. The program will fit your lifestyle. It will be easy, convenient. You won't be hungry. Plus, you'll feel better. You will get in shape, stay healthy and trim.

You will become Smart for Life.

If I can do it, if thousands of my patients can do it, you can too.

Complicating Factors

Despite the exaggerated simplicity presented on television shows like The Biggest Loser, weight gain and loss are actually complicated, multifactorial problems. The solutions to overweight and obesity, *as medical, physical, psychological, economic, and social conditions,* are highly complex. Because of the complexity of obesity, weight loss diets cannot be effective if they are one dimensional, one-size-fits-all. Each individual has his or her own highly personal issues and physiological factors that influence weight gain and loss. There is no simple prescription.

The truth is, it's just not as easy as: eat less, exercise more. As you may remember from my own life experience, if it were that simple, my journey would have been short and sweet, and there would have been no need for Smart for Life.

Take a look at the following list of contributing factors to weight gain. I'm not trying to convince you that weight loss is impossible because it's not. I'm just trying to share with you the complex picture that is the reality of becoming and remaining overweight. We've all got our reasons for gaining too many pounds, and they can be more valid and more complicated than we give ourselves credit for:

Factor #1: Medications that contribute to weight gain include steroids, insulin, antidepressants, and other drugs. (See the drug chart in Chapter 2).

Factor #2: Working too much and/or under great stress can lead to weight gain while sitting in front of a computer for hours at a time can result in an inactive, sedentary lifestyle that supports unhealthy habits and contributes to weight gain and retention.

Factor #3: Vacation can add on the pounds, and most of us go on one at least once a year.

Factor #4: Stress typically encourages over-eating and can affect body hormones that result in extra fat storage. (More on this in Chapter 8).

Factor #5: Poor sleeping habits can lead to weight gain. (More on the link between sleep hormones and fat storage in Chapter 8).

Factor #6: Poor eating habits are the obvious cause, but certain foods (e.g., over-processed, high glycemic index foods) can really contribute to body fat stores while a lack of others (e.g., whole, high fiber foods) can be problematic as well.

Factor #7: Relationships can lead to weight gain (Remember Alan and Jenny?) and breakups can lead to over-eating.

Factor #8: Your social life may be making you fat. If you hang around overeaters and that's the way you socialize, your weight can suffer.

Factor #9: Drinking beer and other alcoholic beverages, even in moderate amounts, can lead to beer bellies and body bloat and eventually to obesity—and other health issues.

Factor #10: Smoking cigarettes is a habit that will kill you, and you should definitely quit, but people who stop smoking do tend to gain weight.

Factor #11: Skipping meals can lead to over-eating and will contribute to metabolic inefficiency.

Factor #12: Fad dieting can cause weight gain as your body's metabolic rate slows and, once the fad is over, weight is regained quickly.

Factor #13: Dining out all the time reduces your ability to control what you are eating. Portion sizes in restaurants tend to be excessively large. They want your business; they don't care if you get fat as long as you come back again and again.

Factor #14: Depression can lead to over-eating, weight gain, and depression about over-eating and weight gain, a vicious circle.

Factor #15: Menopause results in hormonal changes that can cause a wide array of body changes including weight gain.

Factor #16: Aging does lead to a gradual decline in the rate of metabolic activity, making it easier to gain weight over the age of 30 and increasingly difficult to lose weight over the age of 50.

Factor #17: Pregnancy leads to weight gain, obviously, but losing weight after a baby is born can prove difficult due to hormonal—as well as lifestyle—changes.

Factor #18: Miscarriages can cause weight gain from both hormonal changes and emotional influences.

Factor #19: Illness can lead to inactivity, eating unhealthy comfort foods, and over-eating during recovery.

Factor #20: Genes do have an influence on your body size and shape, but you can work within your genetic endowment to attain and maintain a healthy body weight.

It's not so simple, is it? But weight loss is not impossible, either. Keep these factors in mind as you move forward on your journey. Take note of how you are changing your lifestyle and coping mechanisms, moving away from over-eating toward a healthier way of living.

Disorders Causing Weight Gain

Ill health and hormonal imbalances can contribute to the complications of being overweight and obesity. Metabolic factors that contribute to weight gain include fluid retention due to monthly water retention in women of childbearing ages, which can be normal or excessive, as well as certain disorders and dysfunctions that influence fat storage and/or fluid retention.

Before you begin on any weight loss regimen, your doctor will screen you for the following:

* Thyroid problems—Underactive (or hypo-) thyroid can cause fatigue, weight gain and slowed metabolism; proper medication can correct the problem.

*Cushing's syndrome—Excess cortisol, a hormone, causes a stress response that includes storing energy as fat and putting on weight; proper medication can control this disorder.

*Kidney disease—Weight gain that is largely fluid retention may be due to dysfunctions of the kidney.

*Liver disease—Weight gain due to fluid retention can be due to liver dysfunction.

*Adrenal dysfunction—Weight gain may occur due to hormonal imbalances.

*Cardiovascular disease—Fluid retention can also be a sign of weak cardiac function.

*Insulin resistance and type 2 diabetes—Poor insulin response can become a pre-diabetic condition that leads to type 2 diabetes; dietary changes can make a huge difference here.

*Ovarian cysts— PCOS May cause weight gains of 30 pounds or more.

*Depression—Weight gain can accompany periods of depression or chronic anxiety in some people while others may lose weight.

This list of weight influencing disorders should clarify for you why I encourage anyone who is planning to go on a weight loss program first to see a qualified physician. At Smart for Life Weight Management Centers, we conduct thorough exams with our patients who come to us for weight loss aid. That way, if there are any complicating factors, we can identify them before the patient begins the program.

Get Smart and Simplify Your Life

The good news is, once you are on the Smart for Life program, your life should actually begin to simplify. The complicating factors of being overweight or obese will become a thing of the past. Like your diet, you will become healthier. Your life will be more organic, natural, rich in simple pleasures. This is part of the joy of being Smart for Life.

Being healthy in and of itself can simplify your days. No need to remember to take your pills. No time wasted in hospital waiting rooms, emergency rooms, and outpatient clinics. No need to file reams of insurance paperwork. You should discover you are able to spend a lot less time conducting these stressful, complicated activities.

When you eat Smart, you have better energy, and your senses are sharpened. Life comes into keener focus. You can taste the real flavors of natural foods. You may smell the roses. You'll find yourself making time to appreciate the great outdoors, enjoying the spring air, the summer skies, the autumn leaves, the winter chill. You'll be savoring each meal and snack as you eat them, no longer wolfing your food mindlessly. Your mind is freed from worrying about your body and health, no longer bogged down with the old concerns and guilt surrounding your diet. You've freed up your time and energy, too, from the illnesses and weight-related issues that dragged you down. You'll find you have more time and energy to enjoy your family, friends, work, and home life.

This is the joy of simple, Smart living at a healthy weight.

I doubt you need any more encouragement from me at this point. But just in case you need one final push to convince you to embark on and stick to the Smart for Life program, I am including in this chapter some of the massive amount of impressive science that supports the link between eating Smart, maintaining a healthy weight, and living a long and healthy life.

But first, you might want to read about how Jack G. changed his health and his life when he chose Smart for Life.

Jack G.

"For my son's 18th birthday, I asked him to choose a special activity we could do together. He chose skydiving," Jack G. recalls.

At the time, Jack was excited. Jump out of a plane with his son? Hey, why not? The idea sounded great. "But once I looked into skydiving, I found I couldn't do it because I was over the weight limit," Jack says now.

Jack felt dejected. And embarrassed. But his feelings morphed into something else, and he found himself motivated. He had the skydiving bug. He really wanted to have that amazing experience, and he didn't want to disappoint his son. Besides Jack knew he had to lose weight. He suffered from sleep apnea and was on medication for asthma and high blood cholesterol. He was only middle-aged, and already he was totally out of shape.

Jack signed up at a Smart for Life Weight Management Center near his home in Quebec. He started on the program and liked it. He wasn't hungry, and he felt better, healthier.

Before six months passed, Jack G. reached his weight goal. He'd dropped almost 60 pounds.

And he soon discovered he felt better than ever. He looked fit, and he slowly increased his physical activity until he felt fit. He was sleeping better because his sleep apnea had greatly improved. His asthma symptoms were completely gone, so he no longer needed medication. He had more energy. He was able to cut his cholesterol medication prescription dose in half.

"I feel 20 years younger and can maintain rigorous sport activity," Jack reports now. "Basically, I shaved off 20 years and improved my general health."

Friends and family, including Jack's son, tell him, *You're my hero. Keep up the good work.*

Jack G. wants to lose more weight so he can stop taking his cholesterol medication.

After that, the sky's the limit!

Obesity is a serious medical problem in the US and other developed countries. The global threat is growing worse; an increasing number of people are overweight and obese. The problem is spreading into less developed nations as well.

In the US, the number of obese children and teens has tripled since 1980. This means our kids are exposed to all the dangerous health risks associated with being obese for more years than they would be if they stayed fit until adulthood. Fat kids are unhealthy kids and will be seriously unhealthy adults unless they lose weight, which is more difficult for anyone who has been overweight as a youth.

Obesity significantly increases the risk for serious chronic diseases and contributes overall to mortality. Fat people suffer from more illnesses, and their life span is shorter than their healthy weight peers. Do we want to be forced to deal with the following diseases, all of which are associated with excessive body weight? Do we want our kids to have to do so?

*Diabetes, type 2 diabetes, insulin resistance

*Heart disease, elevated blood pressure, elevated blood lipids, metabolic syndrome

*Pulmonary embolism, stroke

*Cancer (certain cancers are associated with diet, obesity, and over-eating, including breast, prostate, colon)

*Polycystic ovarian syndrome

*Gastro-esophageal reflux disease

*Fatty liver

*Hernia

*Erectile dysfunction

*Urinary incontinence

*Chronic renal (kidney) failure

*Osteoarthritis, gout

*Gallbladder disease

*Sleep disorders including sleep apnea

*Increased susceptibility to viruses, reduced immune function

*Allergies, asthma, food allergies and intolerances

*Depression

Note that some of the above ills are also contributing factors to being overweight and obese. See the vicious circle? You are fat so you get sick; you are sick so you gain more weight.

The best solution for avoiding the vicious cycle of chronic illness is to *prevent these diseases in the first place*. This means getting fit and staying fit as early in life as possible. For your kids, that means right now. And for you, that means right now, too. Whatever age you may be, the maxim for getting in shape is: better late than never. Most certainly, keeping your kids fit will help them to avoid the preventable diseases on the above list.

Second best solution for dealing with these chronic diseases is to reduce their impact by losing excess weight and getting back in shape. Staying in shape will improve your overall health, allowing you to reduce or eliminate medications while enhancing the quality of your life. This holds true for your kids as well.

At Smart for Life Weight Management Centers, we see some very unhappy people who come in to the clinics leaning heavily on walkers, short of breath, suffering from arthritis, back pain, insulin resistance, cardiac disease, and diabetes. We see patients who can hardly walk, who can't sleep through the night, who have no sex life, who suffer from suicidal thoughts. We see people, nice people, who are discriminated against because of their weight and, despite the best qualifications, are unemployed. We hear about some really sad weight-related family issues, and our nicest patients commonly admit to a lack of self-love.

This would be overwhelmingly troubling if we did not see so many of our patients succeed. But we have been able to observe thousands of people who have become Smart for Life. We've watched with amazement as these determined individuals turned their lives around, throwing away walkers, finding love, getting new jobs, going back to school, learning how to live again. We've heard stories of patients who asked their doctors if they could reduce or eliminate prescription medicines then found they felt better than they had in years. We've watched as some of our fattest patients trimmed down and transformed themselves into long-distance runners, martial arts experts, body builders, skydivers.

If they can do it, you can, too.

The Western Diet and Disease

Being overweight can make you unhealthy and prone to diabetes, cardiovascular disease, and other serious illnesses, but *eating the Wrong Foods can make you sick even if you are not fat.* This is why the Smart for Life program advocates eating healthy, natural foods for your entire life not just while you are losing weight. And that's why the program is called Smart for Life not Smart Just for Now, but Smart forever.

Scientific and medical studies from around the globe have exposed the truth about the American way of eating: it is making us sick. We have spread our fast food chains and our burgers and fries, our boxed sugary cereals and microwavable convenience meals to the rest of the world, making the Western diet a way of life in many developed countries. Yet, numerous studies show that people who eat a typical Western diet have a higher risk of developing a variety of chronic diseases.

The Western diet has been linked to metabolic syndrome and

cardiovascular disease. Metabolic syndrome is the name for a cluster of symptoms that predispose people to cardiovascular disease. The symptoms include a large waist circumference, high blood pressure, high fasting blood sugar levels, insulin resistance, low levels of HDL ("good") cholesterol, and high triglycerides. The American Heart Association advises us that the typical Western diet may lead to stroke as well as heart disease.

The Western diet is the root cause of these and other chronic diseases. Also known as the Standard American Diet (SAD is not a bad name for it), a regular dietary intake of over-processed foods, fatty sweets, soft drinks, and red meats leads to overweight, obesity, illness, and chronic disease. The typical Western diet includes a lot of refined grains, processed meats, fried foods, whole eggs, and sugary beverages. The SAD does not include enough fresh produce, fish, seafood, low-fat dairy foods, or lean protein. The typical Western diet is far too high in sugar and fat and far too low in vitamins, minerals, fiber, and phytonutrients.

Some researchers believe the Western diet may be responsible for activating specific genes that signal the body to store more fat. This makes sense because, as the Western diet has changed over the past few decades with a significant increase in the consumption of fast foods and junk foods, processed foods high in sugar and unhealthy fats, obesity rates have also risen sharply. It seems that the SAD body is storing more fat than is healthy due to a reliance on the Wrong Foods and/or avoidance of nutrient-rich Smart Foods.

Some studies have implicated the Western diet in the onset of Alzheimer's disease. It appears that Alzheimer's may be promoted by insulin resistance, inflammation, and other factors associated with dietary imbalances. And there appears to be a link between obesity at mid-life, metabolic syndrome and the risk of late-life dementia.

Here's a shocker: the Western diet may be contributing to the sharp increase in the incidence of autism and learning disorders. Mothers with pre-pregnancy obesity have an increased likelihood of giving birth to a baby with an autism spectrum disorder, according to some researchers. There also appears to be a significant correlation between pre-pregnancy obesity and the risk of developmental delays in children. Other studies link obesity in kids with allergies, asthma, and early puberty. And the typical Western diet is at the root of the overweight and obese citizens of our modern society, from youth to old age.

Although these diet-disease links are not proven, the negative influence on overall health of a low nutrient, high fat, sugar rich diet full of artificial ingredients, additives, and preservatives is indeed certain. The evidence is in: eating the typical Western diet is not the way to achieve good health. At both ends of life's spectrum as well as all through the middle years, eating right is essential to optimal health. At any age, eating a diet emphasizing all the Wrong Foods in place of Smart Foods can predispose us to illness and disease.

Eating Less and Living Longer

Scientists and researchers have been aware for many years that animals fed on a high nutrient, low calorie diet will live significantly longer than their peers. Over the years, the life span of a variety of animals—from insects to lab rats to dogs and monkeys—has been expanded significantly using reduced food intakes.

Long-term studies with humans on high nutrient/reduced calorie diets, however, are rare. It's almost impossible to record a person's dietary intake from birth or youth through their entire lives and even more difficult to find people who will actually adhere to a specific diet for much of their lives. But nutrition researchers do believe there is enough evidence to suggest that *eating lesser amounts of largely high-quality foods will improve health, delay aging, and increase the chances for living a long and healthy life.*

Long-term caloric restriction along with optimal nutrient intake has been shown to improve cardiac function and decrease inflammation. Obese and overweight individuals tend to have low-grade chronic inflammation in the body, and this condition leads to a variety of age-related disorders including premature aging and early death. A diet that is nutritionally rich but low in calories will reduce inflammation, thereby improving heart function, overall health, and longevity.

Currently, there is a lot of speculation and much heated discussion among scientists and medical researchers on the topic of reduced calorie diets as a means for slowing the aging process. The jury is not in yet, but I am one of a growing number of health professionals who believe that there is adequate evidence to support the high nutrient/reduced calorie diet as part of an anti-aging lifestyle.

For this reason, among others, the Smart for Life program encourages you to adopt the habit of consuming less food while choosing more healthy food. Smart Foods are naturally high in nutritional value for the calories they provide. You get the most bang for your buck when you choose Smart Foods. A lifetime of doing so will make you feel better, look younger, and live longer.

Eating Smart for the Planet

We think of ourselves as consumers because that's how the food industry has trained us to behave. We are passive in that way, allowing the big food corporations to dictate to us what our appetites should be. This is not good for us, and ultimately it's also bad for the planet.

I think about this subject a lot. I've got kids, and I want them to be able to live in a healthy world that is not too polluted with plastic, garbage, and toxic waste. And personally, I don't want to feel like I've left the planet in worse condition than I found it when I arrived.

So I've been wondering: what if we began to think of ourselves as world citizens instead of consumers? What if we all simply stopped eating the junk, the over-processed and over-packaged Wrong Foods that take up so much space and use up so many resources here on Mother Earth?

Think about it: overly processed foods have a big carbon footprint and a major environmental impact. Think of how these foods are made, creating pollution and wasting resources, adding to the plastic that is not degrading in our dumps and is sucking up the oxygen in our oceans. The production of over-processed foods poisons the environment with petroleum-based additives and packaging materials. Think of all the animals that must be slaughtered to feed our fast food habit. Imagine all the bags and bottles, boxes and cans of shelf-stable foods that are shipped and trucked around the globe. Imagine all the feed lots for animals, the acres of pesticide-saturated land used to grow apples and potatoes just to create the menu items served at fast food restaurants. Then multiply the waste this must create by the huge number of fast food and shelf-stable food products available today. It's mind-blowing. Our junk food habit is taking up too much space on a crowded and increasingly damaged planet.

If we purchased fewer fast and convenience foods, we would not only save on packaging material waste, but we could help reduce the global impact of the production of all these foods. The typical supermarket of the 1960s wowed shoppers as it expanded along with the growth of the modern food industry, offering hundreds of different foods. At today's supermarkets, we may select from 30,000 foods—or more! Do we really need all those food products to choose from?

The wide variety of over-processed foods available to consumers has increased profits for the big food companies, but our health has declined while our waistlines have ballooned. Plus, the garbage we are creating with our appetites for over-processed convenience foods is extensive. And unnecessary.

When I think about this subject, I'm glad I created Smart for Life. Our packaging leans toward green, and the amount you would use in a full day on the Smart for Life program would be less than half the packaging of one typical fast food meal. Plus, our food products are healthy and natural. Being on the Smart for Life program encourages us to eat less, eat better, eat Smart—for our bodies and for the planet.

Losing weight in and of itself can be good for the planet because you are consuming less food, consuming fewer of the most resource-wasting products, and consuming less medical care. You are not going to the drive-thru as often because you are making simple meals at home. You are not buying all those plastic bottles, the Styrofoam containers and plastic bags because you are eating natural, whole foods. You may be walking more and driving less. You're healthier so you are no longer such a drain on the medical system.

Studies show that one-fifth of US energy consumption is used for food production and food transportation. If we eat less to lose weight, we cut down on energy use. By eating less, we can have a significant impact on fuel consumption. If we eat significantly less, the reduction in energy use can be significant, too.

Worldwide, agriculture accounts for around twenty percent of greenhouse gas emissions. Carbon dioxide, methane, and other greenhouse gas emissions are cut back if we lose weight and eat less.

What if everybody in the developed world decided to be an environmentally conscious citizen rather than a passive consumer? *What if we all simply ate less?* Public action of this sort could have a dramatic positive effect on global climate change, energy issues, and world health.

Think about it: eating less could make you healthier. It might help you to live longer. By eating less, you are contributing to the health of the planet. Plus, you lose weight. How can you go wrong here?

Then there is this fact: eating natural, healthy foods has a positive impact on you, your weight, and on the environment. When more and more citizens demand natural, healthy foods, this is good for the planet. Foods made without pesticides and additives, organic foods made without GMOs, are better for us and for Mother Earth. This is why the Smart for Life program includes only healthy, natural foods—better for you, better for your family, better for the planet.

Just so you know, the organic, natural foods of the Smart for Life program make the weight loss method unique. Other weight loss programs do not offer dieters organic foods and healthy natural products. In fact, the organic basis of the program is what draws many people to Smart for Life. People like Suzanne T.

Suzanne T.

She needed to lose more than 70 pounds, but diets didn't work for Suzanne T. She had tried them all without success. She would look at herself in the mirror and get psyched to lose weight. But then she always got hungry and went off the diet plan. She didn't like what she was eating when she was on a diet. The food was full of preservatives; it was unnatural. She always felt tired and unhealthy when she was dieting.

Then Suzanne found out about Smart for Life. She liked the idea of a diet that was mostly organic and composed of natural foods. She liked that the program sounded as if it would fit in with her hectic lifestyle. So Suzanne T. started on Smart for Life.

"I liked the taste of the food I was eating, and I liked knowing that I was consuming foods that are 60% organic without any preservatives," Suzanne says. "That assured me that I was giving my body the best quality nutrition it deserves." She liked how the six daily meal replacements "worked so perfectly in my schedule. It was so easy." She didn't feel hungry, and she had plenty of energy.

She liked Smart for Life so she stuck with it. "My metabolism was consistent throughout the day, and I never felt hungry or sluggish. The weight just kept melting away."

After 10 months on the program, Suzanne had lost more than 70 pounds. She looked and felt fabulous. "Even my skin is healthier looking," she told me.

Suzanne has maintained her weight loss. Whenever holidays and special events lead to overindulgences, "I get back to eating Smart for Life cookies, which has become a way of life for me," she reports. "I've learned from being on the program for so many years that it is a *lifestyle change for life* not just for the period of time until you reach your weight goal."

Suzanne's life has certainly changed since she altered her lifestyle. "No one believes that I'm 53. Most people guess that I'm in my 30s. I get compliments all the time on my figure, and people ask me how I stay so trim. I rave to them about Smart for Life: I'm such a fan!"

Last time I talked to her, Suzanne was planning her wedding. After she'd lost 75 pounds, she'd splurged on a lovely dress. "I bought a white gown that I only wore once. It's a size two. It's been three years, and it still fits beautifully. I am wearing that gown on my wedding day!"

How exciting! I had to agree with Suzanne T. when she said, "The Smart for Life weight loss management system transformed me and my life!"

Believe it or don't, I learned very little about nutrition while I was in medical school. At the time, physicians in training were not required to take classes exploring the link between diet and disease. Like most doctors, I rarely asked a patient about what he or she was eating on a regular basis, and I wasn't too aware of the kind of diet (i.e., junky) I was consuming myself.

But when I had my own great awakening and began to understand the major influence exerted by our food intakes on our overall health, I changed my perspective on nutrition. I realized how important diet was for good health as well as proper weight. And I began a lifelong study of nutrition science, bariatrics or weight loss medicine, diet and disease.

Now, of course, I am keenly aware of what my patients are eating and of my own dietary intakes. A person's nutritional status is a primary factor in determining his or her state of health. *Diet is one of the factors in health care over which we have control.* Like daily activity, avoiding cigarettes, and not drinking alcohol to excess, our dietary intakes are within our power to change and improve. I see this as a matter of life or death because a person's diet can make the difference between living a long and healthy life and being sickly and/or experiencing a premature demise.

Weight control, too, is a health care factor over which we can exert personal control. Losing weight while including adequate nutrients in your diet can improve your health in a variety of ways. Changing your metabolism so that the body works more efficiently will alter the tendency to store excessive body fat. This will result in a healthier, leaner body for life.

Adequate nutrition is key to weight control. Optimal diet is essential for health and longevity. You've got to eat Smart for life to be fit for life.

But you know most of this already from reading the previous

seven chapters. You also understand that nutrition and bariatrics are complex subjects, the science complicated and controversial. I too have trouble understanding all of the research because much of it is based on intricate systems of physiology, genetics, biochemistry, statistics, and epidemiology, which is the study of population groups. I have to study the studies, carefully screening the research and reading between the lines. I always look at who is funding the research. For example, if a study that says sugar is good for you has been funded by some giant breakfast cereal company, well, I have my doubts about that particular piece of so-called evidence.

Personally, I like epidemiological research reports because these studies tend to include large groups of people who are followed for long periods of time. Small studies on animals like lab rats don't impress me as much. But I find contemporary scientific research on diets, dietary factors, nutrients, and the influence on body weight, weight loss, health, and disease to be fascinating. For this reason, I am sharing some of what I have discovered with you here in this chapter.

Because the material is complex and because there is so much of it, I have selected some topics I think you might find especially interesting and pertinent. At this point, you are on the Smart for Life program, and you know enough about the role of diet in weight control and overall health to serve as a solid foundation for making wise food choices. If you flunked biology in high school, you might not want to read this chapter. If medical terminology makes you faint, you can flip to the next chapter right now. But if you are intrigued with medical and nutritional research like I am, read on.

The Caveman Survival Mechanism and You

When our primitive ancestors needed to eat, they didn't have the option of drive-thru burgers or microwaved breakfast pastries. Early humans had to hunt down their food and kill it. This requires a significant expenditure of energy. Gathering wild grasses, berries, ground nuts, and weeds to supplement one's fresh kill takes a lot of energy, too. This explains why it is probable that prehistory's men and women were not obese. They had no leather couches and TV sets, no supersized fast foods and soft drinks.

Lucky them.

What they did have were extended periods of starvation. Winter in most places meant heavy snow and frozen bodies of water, plant food under ice, and hibernating wildlife. To outlast the annual winter season as well as periods of heavy rainfall, drought, and natural disasters, the early humans who survived had bodies that could store up extra energy as fat during the good times when food was plentiful. That way, when food was scarce, the early humans could survive by relying on their stored body fat for energy.

The caveman survival mechanism: we inherited it from our ancestors. If not for this fat storage ability, obesity would not be a problem today. But then again, we would not be here.

It was this ability to store fat that allowed the human species to make it through the tough times. By saving up extra energy for the lean times, humans could hunker down when necessary then reproduce, so that yet another generation might carry on.

That's what fat storage is for: a savings bank for body energy to be used when funds are low and starvation sets in. Fortunately—or maybe, for those of us with weight issues, unfortunately—periods of starvation don't occur on a regular basis anymore for most of us living in developed countries. Meanwhile, our bodies are storing up fat like there's a severe winter right around the corner. Then, if the winter comes, more fat is stored! The local hamburger joint is open, as is the donut shop, the supermarket, the convenience store, and our own kitchen, 24/7: food is available.

Due to thousands of years of programming, the human body is very efficient at storing fat, and the body does not seem to be designed to give up readily those fat stores. Our fat stores were once a matter of life and death: if early humans had shed their stores of energy quickly, before the flood or drought or winter had ended, then the population itself would not have survived, and we wouldn't be here in our

Lazyboy chairs, watching the news and snacking.

You can see why it is easier to gain weight than it is to lose it. Our genetic programming was designed to enable us to pass on our genes, which means we need to survive when times are tough. Does this mean our genes are making us fat?

Yes and no.

Food and Your Genes

Our genes form the template upon which we build our lives. Genes are the blueprint that gives rise to the genetic expression of who we are as individuals. Our genes are the potential for our future selves.

Although we may be born with genes that predispose us to weight gain or fat storage in specific areas, we do not have to express this in our physical selves. We do not have to become as fat as our mothers or fathers, grandparents or siblings. We can make choices with or within our environment—diet, lifestyle, activity, etc.—that will influence our genetic expression and create an alternate self.

In other words, our genes can make us fat but only if we let them by making Wrong Food and lifestyle choices.

The same is true for the influence of our genes on health and disease. Our genes do play a role in defining our risks for inheriting many different diseases, including diabetes, heart disease, and certain cancers. But this does not mean we are fated to die from a chronic disease simply because our ancestors did so. *Healthy aging is controlled by how we communicate with our genes through our diet and lifestyle.*

What does this mean? According to the newest research in molecular biology and ongoing studies at the Human Genome Project, we each have a say in what will happen to us as we age. We can communicate with our genes, in a sense, by providing our cells with the nutrients and other factors they need to function optimally. In doing so, we send to our genes positive messages that result in good health. If, on the other hand, we are eating mostly junk lacking in nutritional value, we will send to our body cells the kind of negative messages that result in poor health and, typically, being or staying overweight.

We as individuals are not simply the reflection of our genes or what scientists call our "genotypes." Our individual selves are also determined by environmental influences that help to create a specific physical, biochemical, and physiological makeup called a "phenotype." There's more to you than your blueprint. There are all of the choices you make when you build the foundation, add on the floors, design and redesign the interior and exterior of your body and your life. Your phenotype includes who you are, what you look like, how your body functions, and what diseases you might have.

Thus, *you can control your genes by controlling your environment.* You can get the most from your genetic blueprint, improving the ways your genes function to enhance your body and positively impact your state of health and wellness.

So, if you choose to, you may express your own phenotype at the optimal level within the genetic factors you inherited. In this way, you may realize your full potential. This means you *can* be trim, healthy, and long-lived *if you work at it.*

The newest science indicates that our genes do not, in and of themselves, cause all disease. Instead, most disease results when we follow a lifestyle that alters the expression of our genes, turning on and off certain genes that allow diseases to be expressed. "Bad" genes do not always cause disease, but when an individual is in a toxic environment, disease may be expressed. Bad habits turn on bad genes and turn off "good" genes, and a toxic environment does the same thing. Environment and lifestyle can determine whether a gene is being expressed or not. *Thus, it is the risk that is inherited, not the disease.*

Your phenotype—who you are—is determined by the way you live, and have lived, and will live. Your phenotype is created by your genetic risk plus what you do with your life. You can modify your phenotype and the expression of your genetic inheritance. You can do this by eating Smart and living Smart.

This is exciting stuff! Although this does not mean we can avoid all disease and live forever, new studies on genes and genetic expression indicate that we have a lot more control over our health than we might have believed.

Not all genetic characteristics are capable of modification through diet, of course. You can't modify your eye color by eating more greens, for example. But a host of genetic characteristics may be influenced by nutrition and lifestyle factors.

It is true that you may be more susceptible to chronic diseases due to inherited factors including individual digestive function, organ health, and unique sensitivities to foods. If this is so, you will want to make sure your diet is optimal so that you achieve and maintain the healthiest body possible. Because you can optimize your genetic blueprint using those factors you can control.

For example, you can increase the fiber in your diet to decrease your risk of colon cancer. This is especially important if colon cancer has been diagnosed in members of your family. Dietary fiber turns off the bad genes that are responsible for colon cancer. This is just one example of the influence of diet on genetic expression.

The foods and nutrients we come in contact with every day are sending chemical messages to our genes and body cells that may lead to an inherited response. Certain genetic characteristics can be expressed, and a disease may be the result. However, *you may choose to limit your exposure to those environmental factors that will lead to this undesirable expression.* You might decide to eat Smart Foods, avoid excessive alcohol intake, get fit, stay fit, and make sure your nutrient intake is topnotch.

Poor quality diets that are low in nutrients but high in sugars, unhealthy fats, artificial preservatives and additives, and other toxic substances provide just the kind of environment that fosters the genetic expression of ill health and disease. You can change your genes by choosing different foods to eat, changing the expression of your genes with your diet. You can change how your genes influence your state of health. This means your food selection is extremely important.

Modern nutrition science tells us there are thousands of substances in the foods we eat that can impact our genes and influence our genetic expression. These substances include health-promoting nutrients like proteins, amino acids, omega-3 fatty acids, vitamins, and minerals as well as fibers, phytonutrients, healthy microorganisms, antioxidants, and other positive messengers. There are also negative messengers in food including unhealthy carbohydrates like sucrose, fructose, and other sugars, unhealthy fats, toxins, poisons, bad microorganisms, additives, and artificial chemicals.

All these substances transmit messages to your body's cells, influencing your health and genes. Some help, some hurt. The key to good health is to emphasize the former and reduce the latter.

When you continuously feed your body's cells supersized messages full of disinformation, the result is impaired metabolic function, excessive fat storage, and other genetic expressions of ill health and disease. Certain nutrients and other food substances can increase your chances for a positive expression, however, enhancing weight loss, improving digestion and organ function, and boosting health and vitality. The dietary choices you make can encourage your body to assist you in reaching your genetic potential for longevity. Weight loss can turn off certain bad genes, and healthy diets can turn on genes for longevity.

As this chapter evolves, we'll be taking a look at the molecular substances scientists know about that can provide positive messages versus those imparting disinformation to the body's cells. In the meantime, here's a story about one of my Smart patients you might find helpful.

When you have only 30 (or 20 or 10) pounds left to lose, sometimes those final pounds can prove the most challenging. But once you reach the finish line, you will realize that the journey was worth the effort. Make that final push and get yourself across the goal line. Like Pauline A., you'll be glad you did.

Pauline A.

She really didn't have that much weight to lose.

Pauline A. wasn't super fat; she certainly wasn't obese. But she really wanted to drop those 30 pounds, the same 30 pounds she'd needed to lose the year before and the year before that. The extra 30 pounds made her figure look blah, her clothes look dowdy, and her body feel old and tired. The finicky, sticky 30 pounds had snuck up on her and wouldn't go away, no matter how much she rode her bike and avoided dessert.

"I wanted to lose 30 pounds, but I am not the type of person to be fussing and measuring foods, trying to cook three meals a day," Pauline says. So when she heard about Smart for Life, it "sounded like the easiest way to control my hunger without having to think *diet*."

Intrigued, Pauline looked into the program. "And it turned out to be the perfect meal replacement for my busy lifestyle."

This was great news. At long last, a program she could stick to! Pauline became determined to lose those 30 pounds.

She signed up at a local Smart for Life Weight Management Center where she learned how to spread her food intake over the day, eating more often to avoid hunger and an out of control appetite. She learned about Smart Foods and Wrong Foods, portion sizes and good nutrition, and leading a healthy lifestyle.

In only 14 weeks, Pauline A. lost those 30 pounds. That was easy, right?

One year later, Pauline had regained 10 pounds and was heading back in the wrong direction. This was "from being careless," she admits, and allowing her old habits to take over again.

Disappointed and frustrated with herself, Pauline realized that she had not adopted the Smart for Life program for life but only for a few months. Once she'd returned to her old eating patterns, the weight had piled back on.

Determined this time to achieve permanent weight loss, she went back to Smart for Life. This time, she made Smart Foods and Smart lifestyle choices a way of life. She soon reached her goal weight. And this time, she maintained it.

"Now I stay on the Smart Maintenance plan and eat the cookies," Pauline explains. "I always feel better when I am using the Smart for Life products and following the plan: I have more energy, I'm less bloated, and I'm more confident about being in control of my eating habits."

And the health benefits for Pauline are impressive. "I suffered from migraine headaches every month, headaches that lasted three days, even with medication. I am thrilled to say the diet has cured me of this! I no longer have migraines. I would have to say this has been the best remedy ever." Pauline also was happy to find out that her blood lipids normalized. "I can almost hear my arteries saying *thank you*!"

Pauline likes the Smart for Life lifestyle and how it makes her feel. "My metabolism is functioning better. I feel younger. I feel healthy!" She tells us that staying Smart for Life has made her feel better all day long. She says she no longer wakes up achy and stiff. She says her skin looks firmer and has better color, and she has more confidence. "I keep my overall appearance up better because I feel pretty. My husband is very happy with me, and I feel good when I'm out with him or friends."

Pauline only needed a few months to reach her weight goal. But to remain at her desired weight, and to feel energetic and healthy, she has chosen to stay on the program. Smart for Life is her lifestyle now.

At this point, Pauline's BMI is in the normal range, and her weight is perfect for her height and age. She's healthy, and she feels terrific.

Pauline A. plans to keep feeling and looking good for life.

A hormone produced by special cells scattered throughout the pancreas, insulin is released into the bloodstream and travels throughout the body. Insulin is involved in the metabolism of carbohydrates, fats, and proteins and the regulation of the cells of the body including cellular growth.

Insulin resistance is a condition where the cells of the body become resistant to the effects of insulin. When this happens, the normal response to insulin is reduced so that higher levels of insulin are needed for results to occur. You can see how this would interfere with normal metabolism and cellular regulation.

Insulin helps the body's cells remove and utilize food energy in the form of sugar (glucose) from the blood. This is one way in which insulin controls your blood sugar levels. You eat food, your blood sugar rises, you need insulin to move the glucose into the cells and allow metabolism and energy release to occur.

Insulin has to bind to insulin receptors on the surface of cells. With insulin resistance, cells do not allow the binding to occur. The pancreas then makes more insulin, which increases the level of insulin in the blood. In this way, insulin is available but is not being properly utilized. You can see how this might make you feel tired and unwell. The potential energy from your food intake is being wasted.

Unless you change your diet and lifestyle, insulin resistance continues to increase over time. As long as the pancreas is able to produce enough insulin, blood glucose levels remain normal. However, when the pancreas can no longer produce enough insulin, blood glucose levels begin to rise. At first this is an issue after meals when the highest amount of blood sugar is circulating. Eventually, blood sugar levels remain elevated between meals. At this point, type 2 diabetes is diagnosed. Fat cells do not become insulin resistant but will continue to absorb sugar (glucose), and more and more body fat will be stored.

You may be genetically predisposed to insulin resistance, but your lifestyle can help you avoid expression of the disorder. You can turn off the bad genes and avoid insulin resistance. Eat Smart, avoid refined carbohydrates and high glycemic index foods, avoid weight gain, and stay in shape. If you are overweight, it is essential to change your diet and lose those excess pounds. Insulin resistance can also be triggered by infection or serious illness, certain medications such as steroids, and severe stress.

Insulin resistance precedes the development of type 2 diabetes. Often, an insulin resistant patient will have high insulin levels in the blood, a spare tire or excess fat in the central part of the body, abnormal blood lipids, and high blood pressure. When this constellation of symptoms occur together, metabolic syndrome is diagnosed. The patient is on his or her way to a full-blown case of diabetes along with cardiovascular disease, chronic illness, and premature death. The chance of dying from sudden cardiac arrest is increased significantly.

Insulin resistance works against the breakdown of fat and prevents weight loss. Your body cannot get rid of any stored fat while your insulin levels are too high. When your body is insulin resistant, your metabolism is inefficient, and you will continue to store too much fat.

When insulin in the body is working properly, the release of this hormone after eating will reduce your appetite and stimulate your metabolism. But when insulin is not working properly, you can feel hungry after eating while your metabolism functions inefficiently. For example, you might eat a big, carbohydrate-rich breakfast but find you are hungry by midmorning. Insulin resistance causes hunger and weight gain and, eventually, metabolic syndrome and type 2 diabetes.

Eating Smart can help you with insulin resistance and metabolic inefficiency. Eating smaller meals throughout the day is an effective way to regulate insulin release and blood sugar levels. Avoiding foods that trigger large insulin releases is also effective, which is why Smart Foods are low glycemic index choices. Food with a low glycemic index will not jack up your blood sugar levels nor boost the demand for insulin. Losing weight, exercising regularly but not excessively, and maintaining a low stress lifestyle will help as well. All are part of the Smart for Life program.

When dealing with insulin resistance, my patients find it is simply a matter of time: after a period of eating Smart, blood sugar levels typically balance out. Once people are Smart for Life, insulin resistance disappears. Many of my patients with type 2 diabetes find they are able to be weaned off their medication (with physician supervision, of course). And my patients with metabolic syndrome find their symptoms reduced or completely gone once they lose weight and get fit with Smart for Life.

We add functional ingredients to the Smart for Life products that will help your body maintain blood sugar levels in the normal range. Our special proteins and functional fibers assist in with regulating blood sugars. So does a diet low in sugar and adequate in lean protein and healthy fats. Being thoughtful about food choices is what being Smart is all about.

Fad diets, on the other hand, can mess with your insulin levels and metabolic efficiency. When your body is not obtaining necessary nutrition and adequate energy to function properly, the insulin response may be unbalanced. And fad diets tend to confuse a body's insulin response, resulting in the use of lean body tissue like muscle for energy rather than the burning of body fat stores for the energy you need. This is a dangerous and unhealthy way to lose weight. Be Smart: avoid fad diets.

In these hectic times, and due largely to our reliance on fast food, convenience food, and on-the-go junk, at least one-fifth of the American population is insulin resistant. It is estimated that half of all obese people have this preventable disorder. But here's the happy truth: insulin resistance, metabolic syndrome, and type 2 diabetes are within your control because they are caused by a faulty diet and lifestyle.

You can take control, reverse the damage, get lean and healthy. Fortunately, you're Smart now. So you know what to do to accomplish this.

Leptin Resistance

Another hormone, leptin, may also be playing a significant role in your weight problem.

Leptin is believed to have an influence on weight management, thyroid function, stress, mental agility, inflammation, immunity, reproduction, and cardiovascular health. It is surprising that medical scientists only discovered this powerful hormone in the 1990s. Since that time, study after study has explored the impact of leptin on body weight and human health.

Yet, you might not have heard about leptin before reading *Smart for Life*. There are plenty of physicians who have never heard of leptin either.

Most hormones are released by organs or glands. Leptin is released into the bloodstream by stored body fat. Because this hormone is created in your body's fat cells, this means your fat stores function like an organ—as well as a bank account for energy. This is a relatively new discovery, and it has changed the way medical science looks at body fat and weight loss.

Many people are under the mistaken impression that fat just sits in the body, something to be lugged around and hidden under loose clothing. But fat is active, creating and converting hormones, causing inflammation and other problems. Your body fat is actively contributing to your health issues.

Leptin travels through the bloodstream, informing the brain about how much fat you have stored. This information affects your metabolism, speeding it up or slowing it down, depending on your level of fat storage. Leptin also influences appetite, satiety, and weight gain and loss.

This makes it clear why leptin resistance is a problem: if your brain is not receiving messages from your body fat stores regarding energy needs, appetite and hunger, you will not know when you need to eat and when you should stop eating. Why would you keep eating if you have excess fat stores and you have already eaten enough? Perhaps because you have developed leptin resistance.

When leptin messaging is reduced or blocked, your body responds as if your fat stores are empty and starvation is at hand. Remember the caveman survival mechanism? This is how the primitive body works. Your metabolism slows and is inefficient.

Leptin resistance seems to go hand in hand with over-eating and may be a result of obesity, carrying excess weight, and poor dietary habits. Body fat causes the bad genes to turn on and the good genes to turn off, resulting in leptin resistance. If you are leptin resistant, you may have difficulty realizing you are over-eating. This vicious cycle explains a lot, doesn't it?

If you have excess body fat, you may be creating too much leptin. And if your body has been making too much leptin, you might be leptin resistant.

If you are a food addict, you may be leptin resistant. If you obsess over food and feel like you are always hungry, even after eating, leptin resistance may be at fault. The current popularity of gastroporn may be linked to our problem with leptin resistance.

The key to leptin balance is to eat Smart. You probably knew I was going to say that. Leptin responds to healthy levels of body fat: not too much, not too little. It's a balancing act, like everything else in the body.

I advise my patients who have leptin resistance to eat small meals throughout the day, eat Smart foods, and lose weight. Once leptin resistance disappears, my patients find it easier to regulate their appetites, control their eating, and achieve a healthy weight. They find their metabolism becomes more efficient, and eating Smart becomes a way of life.

We use a functional ingredient called LeptiCore in some of our products. This natural substance assists with leptin resistance, and my patients tell me it helps to curb appetite and control hunger.

Please be wary of marketers who claim they have developed a

leptin drug. No such drug has been manufactured, and it is unlikely that such a medication will be on the market anytime soon. You don't need a drug for leptin resistance anyway. Living Smart will fix your leptin problems the natural way.

Your Nutrient Primer

You must know by now that I firmly believe good nutrition is essential for health, weight loss and maintenance, and longevity. I'm a huge fan of cutting edge and scientifically stringent nutrition research and a big promoter of nutrient-rich Smart Foods and Superfoods. I like to know what's in the food I'm eating and the role it plays in my body and health.

Now, to ensure that you understand what makes Smart Foods so great and Wrong Foods so detrimental to your health, I'm providing you with this nutrient primer. The science of nutrition is vast and complex, so this primer is just a brief summary of some of the most salient points. Read it if you want to learn a little more about the foods you are eating and the foods you aren't eating anymore. Once you know your nutrition facts, it's difficult *not* to eat Smart.

Carbohydrates:

Carbohydrates ("carbs") are sugars that come in a variety of forms and are found in a variety of foods. Carbs provide the body with fuel for energy and body function. But carbs are not all created equal.

Most food carbs are sugars, starches, and fibers. Sugars are simple molecules while starches and fibers are, basically, chains of sugar molecules. These chains can be long or short, straight or wildly branched. Some sugars you may be familiar with include table sugar (sucrose), fruit sugar (fructose), corn sugar (including high fructose corn sweeteners), dextrose, and glucose.

During digestion, carbs are broken down into sugar components small enough for absorption into the bloodstream. The sugars are all converted to glucose to allow for transportation by the bloodstream. It is glucose that can be used by the body's cells for energy.

Fiber, however, is different. Fiber is a good carb. Fiber cannot be broken down by the digestive system into sugar components for conversion to glucose. In fact, fiber cannot be digested, so it passes through the digestive system intact. Water soluble fibers will bind to fats and help reduce fat absorption while insoluble fibers promote good gastrointestinal function. Soluble fibers also help control hunger and keep blood sugar levels steady. Fiber is great stuff.

We should consume at least 30 grams of fiber a day, but most Americans don't even get half that amount in their diets. On the Smart for Life program, this will no longer be a problem for you. The diet plan is rich in fibrous foods like veggies and flaxseed, plus we've added some super-fibers to our products.

The best food sources of carbs have fiber, micronutrients and/or phytonutrients. The worst food sources of carbohydrates—bad carbs—are mainly sugar that are quickly digested and converted to glucose. Bad carbs—refined foods, soft drinks, highly processed starches, and sweets—contribute to weight gain, interfere with weight loss and lead to insulin resistance, diabetes, and heart disease.

Fructose, in the form of high fructose corn syrup and other corn sweeteners, is perhaps the worst carb. Small amounts of fructose are found in vegetables and fruits in conjunction with fiber and nutrients. The natural fructose in produce is not unhealthy and was once an important dietary constituent.

Historically, high-fructose fruits ripened and were available just before the winter set in. Thus, nature provided a ready source of fructose to be converted by the body to stored fat, important for those who would soon suffer the scarcity of long winters with little to eat. This once lifesaving contribution to the human diet is no longer necessary in developed countries. However, now we are consuming high-fructose produce year-round. And, when added to processed foods in huge amounts, fructose sweeteners overwhelm the body's capacity to process the sugar. This can be a threat to health.

Unlike other sugars, fructose is processed in the liver. When too much fructose is consumed, the liver creates fats and triglycerides. High levels of certain fats and triglycerides in the blood is a risk factor for heart disease.

Studies show that fructose intake can upset the appetite control mechanism, resulting in lack of satiety. By spiking insulin, fructose intakes lead to more eating, and more hunger. As increasing amounts of fructose have been added to more and more processed foods over the past few decades, this dietary change has gone hand in hand with a boom in obesity, notably in kids. There is mounting evidence that excess fructose consumption leads to over-eating, becoming overweight, insulin resistance, and type 2 diabetes. This would not come as a surprise to anyone who understands nutrition.

Here's the deadly cycle in summary:

A high carb diet with fructose and fructose sweeteners—>hunger, over-eating—>liver processes excess triglycerides—>elevated blood triglycerides—> excess fat storage—>insulin resistance, leptin resistance—>weight gain, increasing insulin resistance, appetite increases—> metabolic syndrome—>type 2 diabetes, heart disease—>weight gain, illness—>premature death

So why are we consuming so much fructose? Because it's cheap and sweet, so the food industry is adding it to practically everything they process. High fructose corn syrup is inexpensive and abundant due to the massive corn subsidies provided to farmers by the US government.

This is one of the reasons I'm so down on the food industry with all of their over-processed foods. Apparently, they value their own profits over the health and well-being of world citizens, including kids. That means the discretion must be ours: read labels and avoid foods made with fructose, corn sweeteners, and the healthy sounding "fruit juice concentrates" that are also high in fructose.

Don't buy any processed foods that contain fructose. Vote with your wallet: if you stop buying these unhealthy products, the food industry will eventually stop making them. Due to public protest, some manufacturers are already responding by removing high fructose corn syrup from their product recipes.

Carbohydrate intake elevates blood sugar levels, so carbs can be high glycemic foods. The glycemic response, however, depends on both the form and amount of carbs consumed.

The glycemic index is a numerical ranking for carbs based on the rate of conversion to glucose within the body. The glycemic index uses a scale of 0 to 100 with higher values given to foods that cause the most rapid rise in blood sugar. Pure glucose is ranked at 100. While sugar-rich foods tend to rank high on the index, some starchy carbs also result in a rapid glycemic response. This is why the Smart for Life diet plan does not include potatoes and sweet potatoes, rice, bread, pasta, and the like.

As you may recall, foods that cause a rapid and significant glycemic response may cause a brief elevation in mood and energy followed by the undesirable cycle of increased hunger, lack of energy, plus weight gain and fat storage. Because of these and the associated health issues, I advise my patients to avoid all high glycemic index foods while losing weight. Once you are on Smart Maintenance, you might want a small taste once in a while, like some cake on your birthday. Once you are fit, however, I will warn you that your body will become more sensitive to sugar-rich foods and less tolerant of high glycemic carbs. A little bit will be plenty.

Size is important, too: medical scientists refer to the quantity of carbs and their effect on the bloodstream as the "glycemic load." The mathematical formula used by nutritionists to calculate the glycemic load is: GL = Glycemic Index/100 x Net Carbs with Net Carbs being equal to the total carbohydrates in grams minus the grams of dietary fiber. All you need to remember is this: the higher the glycemic load, the worse the effect on your blood glucose. This is why a supersized soft drink, for example, provides a double whammy: all that sugar in one sitting: both a high glycemic index and a huge glycemic load.

But it is simple to adhere to a diet that minimizes the glycemic load: choose no-sugar or unsweetened foods and eat very small amounts of any carbohydrate-rich foods. Be sure to include plenty of fibrous foods in your meals and snacks. In other words, eat Smart.

Protein:

In the same way that carbs are made up of sugar molecules, proteins are composed of amino acids. Some amino acids can be manufactured by the body; others must be consumed in foods. The amino acids we need to get from our diets are called essential amino acids.

For health reasons, we should obtain at least 8 grams of protein per 20 pounds of body weight per day. Protein in amounts less than this can cause the body to break down lean body tissues like muscles to obtain the amino acids required for proper function.

However, protein needs vary from person to person. Kids need more protein because they are growing. Pregnant women need more protein, and people who are recovering from illness and surgery may need more as well. Inadequate protein intakes will cause muscle wasting, reduced immune function, growth failure, and organ damage.

The protein you consume is broken down by the body into amino acids, which are then used to build and repair tissue. Protein can be found all throughout your body—in your hair, skin, nails, muscles, bones, and other tissues. Protein creates the enzymes that are required for the chemical processes of the body, and the hemoglobin that carries oxygen in your bloodstream contains protein.

Unlike some other nutrients, amino acids are not stored by the body. This means you need adequate supplies every day. You need to eat foods that provide your body with protein from all of the essential amino acids on a daily basis.

Animal protein foods—meat, fish, seafood, dairy food, eggs—

have all of the essential amino acids you need. Vegetable protein foods—legumes, nuts, vegetables—tend to be low in one or more essential amino acids but higher in fiber and phytonutrients, so I encourage my patients to include both animal and vegetable proteins in their daily diet.

The best animal protein sources are lean chicken and turkey, lean fish and seafood, low-fat or nonfat dairy foods, and egg whites. If you eliminate these foods because you are a vegan, you will have to be very careful to make sure you include adequate protein in vegetable form. This means a lot of soy foods and probably a supplement to ensure adequate micronutrient intake.

Don't get me wrong; I do think a vegetarian diet can be very healthy. But a vegan diet—with no animal products at all—must be precisely planned to be sure it satisfies all of the body's nutritional needs. If you are vegan, be sure to be a Smart vegan. Veganism can be a very healthy way to live.

Note that protein foods have an effect on the appetite control mechanism and contribute to satiety. The albumen in eggs is especially effective. HungerBlock, in fact, is made from egg whites. We add special proteins to some Smart for Life products to help curb appetite. Protein is digested more slowly than carbohydrate, and this helps you to feel full longer. Plus, protein does not boost blood glucose, maintaining a steady blood sugar level, keeping mood and energy consistent and even.

Diets that have adequate protein and are low in high glycemic carbs are believed to reduce the risk of heart disease and diabetes. Such diets also allow for weight loss. Excessively high-protein diets, however, may increase the risk for osteoporosis because calcium must be drawn from the bones to help neutralize or "buffer" the amino acids in the bloodstream. Diets based on red meats and other protein foods high in fat are unhealthy. I'll explain the reasons for this in the next section.

Fats:

Fats are essential to health, and we do need some fat in our diet.

But certain fats are unhealthy while others contribute to good health. You need to be able to tell the difference.

Almost all foods have some fat in them. Ever wonder how they get corn oil out of corn? Vegetables have fat, too. However, the fat found in vegetable foods is insubstantial compared to the amount in meats and other animal foods.

Fat serves as a source of energy. There is fat in your cell membranes, supporting cellular function. Fats can also reduce inflammation—or trigger it, depending on the type of fat.

Fat cannot dissolve in water. To travel through the blood, fat is carried in protein molecules called lipoproteins. These transport molecules include low-density lipoproteins (LDLs or "bad cholesterol") and high-density lipoproteins (HDLs or "good cholesterol").

Cholesterol is a fat-like substance made in the body and obtained through the diet. The body uses cholesterol to make hormones, vitamins, and other vital compounds. Too much cholesterol in the blood is believed to be a risk factor for heart disease. Foods rich in cholesterol—which is not a nutrient because it can be manufactured by the body—include red meats and fatty meats, full-fat dairy products like whole milk and cheese, cream and ice cream, and egg yolks.

For cholesterol sensitive people, blood cholesterol levels rise and fall in relation to the amount of cholesterol included in the diet. Avoiding cholesterol-rich foods can have a substantial effect on the blood cholesterol levels for sensitive people. Other people can eat all the cholesterol-rich foods they want, and their blood levels remain in the normal range. Unfortunately, at this point, there is no way to easily identify responders to dietary cholesterol. For this reason, we keep dietary cholesterol intakes low on the Smart for Life program. This means no red meat, full-fat dairy, or whole eggs.

Low-density lipoproteins (LDL) help to transport cholesterol throughout the body. When there is too much LDL cholesterol in the blood, deposits form in the walls of the arteries. Such deposits—called plaque—can narrow arteries and limit blood flow and may eventually cause a heart attack or stroke. For this reason, LDL cholesterol is often referred to as the bad cholesterol.

On the other hand, some lipoproteins appear to be health supporting. High-density lipoproteins (HDL) scavenge cholesterol from the bloodstream, from LDL, and from artery walls, returning it to the liver for disposal. This is why HDL cholesterol is called the good cholesterol.

The types of fat in the diet, as well as the dietary intake of cholesterol, help to determine the amount of total, LDL, and HDL cholesterol in the bloodstream. Blood triglyceride levels are influenced by dietary intakes, too.

Triglycerides and fatty acids are the small molecules that make up most of the fat we eat. Like glucose from carbs, triglycerides are the form of fat that travels through the bloodstream. But triglycerides are composed of glycerol as well as three fatty acids. And glycerol is converted to glucose in the bloodstream.

Triglycerides and diet are misunderstood. Elevated levels of triglycerides in the blood are due to excess carbohydrate in the diet and not excess fats.

As you know, the body transforms carbohydrates into glucose to be used for energy. Any excess glucose is converted to triglycerides and stored as fat. Some triglycerides will remain in the bloodstream, increasing the possibility of clotting and blockage, which could lead to heart attack or stroke. If you have high cholesterol as well as high triglycerides, your chances of developing heart disease increase significantly.

Anything that increases blood glucose will potentially increase triglycerides, so you should lower your intake of high glycemic and bad carb foods. The more bad carbs you eat, the higher the level of triglycerides in your blood. Fructose especially contributes to increased triglyceride synthesis and a rapid conversion to body fat. An excess of fructose in the diet leads to elevated blood triglycerides and too much stored body fat.

Fats that are saturated contribute to increased LDL cholesterol on the blood while some unsaturated fats may boost blood levels of HDL cholesterol. Unsaturated fats are called good fats, in fact, because they can improve blood cholesterol levels, reduce inflammation, and improve overall health. Unsaturated fats are predominantly found in plant foods like vegetables, nuts, seeds, and the oils made from them. Monounsaturated fats are found in high concentrations in canola and olive oils as well as in avocados, nuts, and seeds. These are healthy unsaturated fats. This is why they are Smart Foods. And this is why Smart food products are made with canola oil.

Omega-3 fatty acids are also healthy fats. You can find omega-3s in abundant amounts in fish and shellfish, flaxseeds, walnuts, and oils such as flaxseed and canola. The three most influential omega-3 fatty acids are alpha-linolenic acid, eicosapentaenoic acid (EPA), and docosahexaenoic acid (DHA). A diet rich in omega-3 fatty acids may help reduce the incidence of cardiovascular disease, type 2 diabetes, and depression and is believed to improve skin, hair, nails, and joint health.

Omega-6 fatty acids are less healthy. These common fatty acids are abundant in refined vegetable oils like corn oil and soybean oil. Our diets tend to have unbalanced fatty acid ratios with too much of the omega-6 fatty acids and not enough of the omega-3 fatty acids. This is because processed foods like junk foods, snack foods, and fast foods tend to be made with soybean oil and corn oil.

Next time you are in a supermarket, take a look at the labels of convenience and packaged foods. You'll notice that most of them list corn oil and/or soybean oil, both high in omega-6 fatty acids. This is why Smart for Life products include ingredients like fish oils, canola oil, and flaxseed, which can help you achieve a healthier fatty acid ratio. And this is why the Smart for Life program includes plenty of fish.

Saturated fats are also known as bad fats. These fats are found in meat and whole-fat dairy products as well as in the coconut oil, palm oil, and palm kernel oil found in many processed foods. (Check processed food labels for these oils too). Saturated fats boost total cholesterol by elevating the bad LDL cholesterol.

Another form of fat is trans fat, what I call evil fat. Trans fats are not found in nature but are formed during food processing. Trans fatty acids are made by heating liquid vegetable oils in the presence of hydrogen gas, a process called hydrogenation. Partially hydrogenated vegetable oils are more stable and less likely to spoil when food is preserved rather than eaten fresh. These oils can withstand repeated heating, making them ideal for frying fast foods.

Thus, these evil fats are convenient for the food industry. But these particular processed fats are bad for our health: Trans fats raise the bad LDL and lower the good HDL. They contribute to inflammation, heart disease, and possibly other ills.

Common food sources of trans fats include margarine, commercially prepared baked goods and snack foods, a wide variety of processed foods from crackers to spreads as well as fast foods and fried foods prepared in restaurants.

Check food labels for trans fats. New labeling laws make listing trans fats mandatory.

Be Smart: Avoid trans fats entirely.

Micronutrients:

Another name for vitamins and minerals, micronutrients are essential nutrients that play a variety of important roles in growth and development, health and longevity. A diet that does not include adequate amounts of micronutrients will lead to illness, chronic disease, and a shortened life span.

We need to consume a diet with the proper amounts of the following vitamins and minerals. Note that excessive intakes of micronutrients in the form of mega-supplements can lead to nutrient imbalances. Use of high doses of micronutrients has not been proven to cure disease:

*Vitamins: vitamin A; vitamin B complex including B1 or thiamin, B2 or riboflavin, B3 or niacin, pantothenic acid, B6 or pyridoxine, biotin, folic acid, B12, choline, inositol; vitamin C; vitamin D; vitamin E; vitamin K

*Minerals: calcium, magnesium, phosphorus, potassium, sodium, chloride; trace minerals include chromium, copper, iodine, manganese, molybdenum, selenium, iron, zinc

Phytonutrients:

Phyto is Greek for plant. Phytonutrients are found in a wide variety of plants. There are many phytonutrients that food scientists already know about and others we have yet to discover.

Although phytonutrients may not be essential for life, and therefore you can live without them, nutritionists think they are important enough to be called nutrients. Phytonutrients are believed to play a role in immune function, and by acting as antioxidants, may help to prevent cancer, slow the damage caused by aging, reduce inflammation, and enhance longevity.

The richest food sources of phytonutrients are fruits, vegetables, legumes, nuts, and teas. Some examples of phytonutrients include:

*carotenoids—brightly colored pigments in fruits and veggies, including beta-carotene in carrots, lutein in greens, lycopene in tomatoes, and pink grapefruit

*flavonoids and polyphenols—found in onions, red grapes, strawberries, raspberries, blueberries, cranberries, and certain nuts; quercetin and catechins are common in fruits and vegetables, flavonols in tea and red wine

*plant sterols—found in fruits and vegetables, grains

If it seems like too much of a challenge to keep all this nutrition information straight in your mind, don't worry. The Smart for Life program accomplishes the task for you, providing you with a nutrient rich diet while you lose weight and get fit. Remember to emphasize Superfoods and be sure to include a variety of fresh veggies in your daily diet.

You may want to think of it like this: nutrients are chemical messengers, helping the body to work efficiently and maintain good health. If your nutritional intake is in balance, your body will be healthy. If your daily intake is deficient in nutrients or you have an excessive intake of unhealthy foods, your body will suffer. Being Smart for Life means eating a well-balanced diet that provides adequate amounts of essential nutrients and supports the maintenance of a healthy weight for a long and healthy life.

More on Hormones and Your Weight

In addition to insulin and leptin, there are a number of other hormones that exert an influence on body weight. I want to tell you about a few of them, but keep in mind that the body is a complex machine, so this information has been simplified.

Thyroid hormones control the rate of metabolic processes in the body. When thyroid hormones are below normal, the body slows down and weight gain, among other symptoms, results. Note that in animals, thyroid hormones elevate in the spring and decrease in the autumn. This fact may explain why winter weight gain seems so easy and why weight loss efforts pay off more readily in the spring. In general, sunlight influences body weight by stimulating the metabolic rate and increasing the production of certain hormones.

Some lesser known hormones that are important in weight control are cortisol, peptide YY, cholecystokinin (CKK), ghrelin, and neuropeptide Y (NPY). All of these hormones are secreted by cells in the gastrointestinal system. In fact, there are more than two dozen hormones secreted by the gut. Many of these hormones are also secreted by the brain. For this reason, medical researchers sometimes refer to the gut as "the second brain."

This is why I am so adamant about food quality: your intestinal system is the first point of contact between any food that you eat and your body. It is a contact point for your body and the outside world. Think of it this way: the intestinal tract is a hollow tube, and whatever is inside this tube is actually outside your body. Your gut is the filter between a world of microbes and your body's organs and tissues.

Your gastrointestinal system is receiving information from the food you eat, passing these messages to your brain and body cells. Hormones are involved; neurochemicals are released. Obviously, we must give our bodies the right messages to be lean and fit, healthy and happy.

Abnormal levels of gut hormones—as well as other hormones—have been reported in animals and humans with obesity. Disturbed levels of cortisol and PYY have been linked to disordered eating behaviors and appetite regulation problems.

Cortisol is a stress-related hormone. Elevated cortisol may mean the body is under stress. PYY is released by the intestinal tract after eating has occurred. Larger amounts of PYY are excreted whenever protein is ingested. This hormone acts on the brain to suppress appetite, making it clear why protein—like the egg white in HungerBlock—reduces appetite and helps with weight loss efforts.

CKK is secreted by the gastrointestinal system when food is present and plays a role in digestion and satiety. CKK acts quickly to alert the body to a feeling of fullness while PYY is slower to message the brain. Both of these gut hormones have a faster response time than leptin, which comes from body fat.

Ghrelin is secreted by the stomach when the body feels hungry. Ghrelin acts on the brain to stimulate eating behaviors.

NPY is secreted by the gut, stimulating eating behaviors and contributing to an increase in the storage of food energy as body fat. When secreted by the brain, NPY will block pain signals and contribute to a feeling of calmness.

When you consider the actions of these hormones, you can understand why starvation diets don't work, how eating can become addictive, and how food helps to relieve stress. Our hormones work in conjunction with the brain to coordinate eating, appetite, mood, and satiety. This system can be upset by fad dieting, over-eating, Wrong Foods, and unhealthy food-related behaviors.

Our sleeping patterns matter, too. When we sleep, our hormones are regulated. Insomnia and poor sleep patterns can disturb hormone balance. Disrupted sleep has been linked to changes in circulating leptin and ghrelin. Animals and humans who are sleep deprived have an increased appetite, slowed metabolism, and elevated blood sugar levels. People who subsist on less than five hours of sleep per night are more prone to weight gain and weight related disorders like type 2 diabetes.

More on Your Gut

Here's some surprising information: more than 95% of your body's serotonin may be manufactured in your bowel. This is strange but true. The fact is, the gastrointestinal system has more nerve cells than your spine. Every neurotransmitter found in the brain can also be found in the gut. This is why your digestive system is believed to act like a second brain.

Serotonin is a neurotransmitter with effects on mood, appetite, and eating behaviors. Low serotonin levels can lead to depression while foods—notably carbs—can elevate serotonin in the body and brain. Consistently low levels of serotonin may be associated with addiction, which could mean that one might be addicted to food as a means for mood elevation. Thus, the gut plays an important role in eating behaviors typically attributed to control by the brain.

To keep the gastrointestinal system healthy, it is essential that you understand the role of the bacterial microflora that populate the gut. This subject is not well understood by many people, including physicians. We didn't learn much about this in medical school, but we should have studied gut bacteria and health because it is very important.

Here's a simplified explanation of how it works: in your large intestine and colon, a variety of bacteria are constantly competing for dominance. Some of these bacteria support health, some not. The key to intestinal health is to have enough of the good gut flora to keep the bad flora in check. When the good flora is dominant, your body will digest food properly and eliminate regularly. All's well that ends well, if you know what I mean. If the bad flora is dominant, your body will suffer. You may have diarrhea and/or constipation. You might develop irritable bowel syndrome or other digestive disorders.

Your gut bacteria works to process food while protecting your body from inflammation. Your gut flora helps you to maintain health and immunity from disease. Studies link unhealthy gut flora to allergies and other ills. Recent studies indicate that obesity is associated with imbalance in the normal gut flora.

It's easy to get out of balance. Unhealthy gut flora can become dominant after antibiotic use. Antibiotics will kill intestinal bacteria, including the good bacteria. An imbalance in gut flora can also occur during travel to other countries where the food and water introduce new flora to your system. Contaminated food in restaurants or at home may also introduce bad gut flora into your system, which can lead to an undesirable imbalance. Sometimes an abundance of chlorine in water supplies can lead to an imbalance in gut microflora. Eating a diet of over-processed foods will also result in gut microflora imbalances.

Cultures with a simple diet of unrefined cereals, legumes, nuts, and vegetables have gastrointestinal systems that function better and support healthier intestinal bacteria. People eating a Western diet tend to have less healthy bacteria in the gut and suffer from more health complaints like allergies, inflammation, and obesity. Diets with excessive sugar, fat, and junk and fast foods disrupt the balance in healthy bacteria and allow harmful bacteria to flourish.

The modern Western diet of high-sugar, low-fiber processed foods is contributing to allergies and other problems not seen in those who eat more primitive diets. A steady diet of junk foods alters beneficial gut bacteria, which in turn disrupts normal digestive function.

Fortunately, gut flora can be improved and healthy balance restored rather easily with a Smart diet of fresh foods and the use of probiotics. I recommend probiotics to my patients to help with proper digestion and weight control.

Probiotics are live bacteria, the kind that will thrive in your intestinal system to outcompete the unhealthy microflora. The best food sources of probiotics are fermented dairy products like yogurt and kefir. Some fermented vegetables also contain probiotics including sauerkraut, kimchi, and fermented soy in the form of tempeh, miso, or soy sauce.

Probiotic supplements as tablets, pills, and powders can be purchased in health food stores. Always keep probiotics refrigerated because the microflora is alive and will die without proper storage.

Studies on obese humans have found that their gut flora tends to be unbalanced. This is true in obese children, too. Nutrition scientists believe that improper gut flora may be contributing to weight gain by inhibiting proper digestion and assimilation of nutrients. I agree, and I think that an imbalance in the environment of the second brain leads to weight gain because it also interferes with food messaging and hormonal activity. Immune function in the gut is dependent on proper microflora, and the metabolism of bacteria in the gut influences hormone secretion.

Everything works together in the second brain to support your good health, but you must feed your body what it needs to be fit.

More studies are underway on this fascinating subject, but in the meantime it's Smart to understand the importance of maintaining a healthy gastrointestinal system. Because you now know how the digestive system influences eating behaviors, appetite regulation, body weight, and overall health, it makes sense for you to keep your gut microflora as healthy as possible.

Metabolic Efficiency and Aging

Like a car kept in good running condition, maintaining your body's health will help you live longer. It's that simple. If your car engine is efficient, your classic automobile may still be on the road after decades of use. This is also true for your body's engine. An efficient metabolism contributes to healthy aging and longevity.

In fact, research shows that *a key element in longevity is optimum metabolic efficiency*. This may be achieved through a diet rich in nutrients and low in unhealthy factors and by attaining and maintaining a healthy body weight. Metabolic efficiency is displayed at every level in the body from the body's regulatory systems to all of the organs to each individual cell. The more efficient your metabolism is, the better everything functions and the longer—and healthier—your life will be.

There are many scientific studies exploring the influence of metabolic efficiency on health and longevity. Plus, it makes sense: live healthy, and your body will function more efficiently. If your body runs more efficiently, you'll age more slowly and last longer. Like a well-preserved classic car from the 1920s, you'll still be rolling along at 80, 90, and beyond.

Obviously, our diets play a significant role in achieving metabolic efficiency and encouraging longevity. This is why Smart for Life relies on fresh vegetables, lean protein, and foods that are rich in nutrients, micronutrients, and phytonutrients rather than sugar, fat, or junky calories. A healthy diet will support good health and long life. You should understand the relationship by now.

One more fact that explains how Smart eating contributes to longevity is the following: antioxidants in food may slow aging.

Micronutrients and phytonutrients can serve as antioxidants in the body. The Smart for Life program encourages a generous intake of foods naturally rich in antioxidants. Antioxidants are chemical compounds that inhibit oxidation, the process that causes rust. The more rusty your car gets, the older it looks and the worse it runs. This is true for the human body as well.

Cellular oxidation produces damaging molecules called free radicals. Free radicals are created during everyday living in reaction to normal stresses like sunlight, air pollution, cigarette smoke, and improper diet. A buildup of free radicals contributes to the aging process and to the development of a number of age-related diseases such as cancer, heart disease, and inflammatory conditions like osteoarthritis. Keeping free radical production low reduces cell damage and slows aging.

Antioxidants are abundant in plant foods. Antioxidants include certain vitamins—A, C, and E—and phytonutrients like polyphenols and carotenoids. In the body, these substances work against the rusting process caused by free radicals, preventing damage to cell function. The buildup of free radicals in the body tends to increase as we age. The results are obvious: wrinkling skin, sagging muscles, slowed mental acuity, organ dysfunction, reduced immunity, illness. The older the car gets, the more careful we must be to protect it from rust.

Eating Smart will help. Achieving and maintaining a healthy weight will also contribute to a reduction in free radical formation. This leads to a slowing of the damage caused by aging, including wrinkled skin and other cosmetic effects, and can support the longevity that results from running your body efficiently for the rest of your life.

Eating less food in general helps to limit free radical buildup. Studies on insects, mice, rats, dogs, and other animals show that reduced caloric intakes (with adequate nutrition) can add years to the life span. Medical researchers believe a lifetime of eating well but not over-eating can contribute to metabolic efficiency, reduced free radical production, and optimal cellular function. And longevity. Smart for Life encourages you to eat less, eat Smart, and live long and well.

Bonus Section

"Our bodies are our gardens, our wills are our gardeners."

—William Shakespeare

ThinAdventure Healthy Weight Program for Kids

Today, about one in three American kids is overweight or obese. This is triple the rate from when I was a kid. With good reason, childhood obesity is now the number one health concern of parents in the United States, ranking higher than both drug abuse and cigarette smoking.

Among children today, obesity is causing a broad range of health problems that previously weren't seen until adulthood. These include type 2 diabetes, high blood pressure, and elevated blood cholesterol levels. As you know, being overweight has been linked to higher and earlier death rates in adulthood.

So, will our kids live as long as we do? Maybe not.

One of the most memorable pronouncements regarding the severity of the current childhood obesity epidemic came from former United States Surgeon General Richard Carmona, who stated:

"Because of the increasing rates of obesity, unhealthy eating habits, and physical inactivity, we may see the first generation that will be less healthy and have a shorter life expectancy than their parents."

In addition to the physical health issues, there are serious psychological effects associated with being overweight when young. In general, fat children are more prone to low self-esteem, negative body image, and depression.

Our kids are fat and they are suffering.

When offering a diagnosis of "overweight" in children and

adolescents, it's important to consider both weight and body composition. Among American children ages 2–19, the following numbers are overweight or obese according to the National Health and Nutrition Examination Survey of 2007-2009:

* for non-Hispanic whites, 31.9% of boys and 29.5% of girls

* for non-Hispanic blacks, 30.8% of boys and 39.2% of girls

* for Mexican Americans, 40.8% of boys and 35.0% of girls

These statistics are both disturbing and unnecessary. Our kids don't have to be fat. We can help them become fit and Smart for Life.

Children today must face many obstacles if they are overweight. They get teased and bullied, overlooked by teachers and potential friends, judged and disrespected by teachers and employers. In a culture obsessed with looksism, fat kids have a tough time achieving their potential.

Overweight kids tend to be sicklier than their normal weight peers. Studies show kids who are above the ideal weight for height are more likely to develop chronic diseases like type 2 diabetes, early signs of heart disease like elevated blood lipids and blood pressure, childhood disorders including asthma and other respiratory ills, and a variety of additional health issues.

Take an honest look at your child. *If your kid is overweight or obese, you need to regard their weight as a serious medical issue.*

Like overweight adults, fat kids struggle with emotional issues related to their body size. They may suffer from depression. One of my patients illustrates this point in a way that I will never forget.

Patient Y

When I was a resident working in the ER, a 16 year old girl was admitted. Let's call her Patient Y. This young woman had a huge impact on me. In fact, Patient Y is one of the reasons I am so adamant today that children should not be allowed to get fat. And if they are fat, they should be helped in every way so that they can attain a healthy weight.

The girl came into the ER on a stretcher, bleeding and half-conscious. She appeared to be what we call a suicidal acting out. She had attempted suicide but not successfully. Perhaps she did not really want to die. She had not slashed her wrists deeply enough to actually kill herself. She had used a straight razor to cut herself enough to need some stitches, however, and had taken some kind of pills. Not enough to overdose but enough that we needed to pump her stomach.

We treated her with ipecac to make her vomit then we inserted a tube down her throat into her stomach to clear out the drugs she had swallowed. We stitched up the cuts on her wrists. She was not in danger and rested quietly on a gurney behind a curtain.

At this point, a patient with Patient Y's history would be sent over to the psychiatric ward of the hospital. In a busy ER, the physician on duty will stabilize the patient, do a preliminary diagnosis, and then refer the patient to the appropriate department. There is always another patient waiting, and ER doctors are always in a hurry to get to them.

But for some reason, I was able to spend some time with this girl. I had a few minutes between patients, so I stayed by her side. And we chatted.

I'd begun thinking of her as Patient Y. As in, why was she so profoundly depressed at such a young age?

Patient Y was significantly overweight. Her belly was huge, her legs and arms like thick sausages. Even her pretty face was swollen with excess fat.

I asked her how she was feeling.

She shrugged, her eyes downcast, as if she felt that she did not deserve to receive my concern. Then she took a deep breath and opened up a bit. "I feel awful," she said. "I hate myself."

When I attempted to reassure her that there was no reason to feel this way and that she would get plenty of help on the psychiatric ward, Patient Y gave me a look. Her eyes were red and puffy, but I could see the intelligence in them. And the pain. She told me, "You don't understand. I hate myself, and there's nothing anyone can do. I hate my body. I hate my life. Nobody likes me because I'm fat."

And Patient Y turned her face away from me. She lay on the stiff white sheets, suffering. And she was right: There was nothing I could do. I stood helplessly by her side for a few moments until an orderly came and wheeled her away to the psyche ward.

I never saw her again.

At the time, I was young and did not have children of my own. But I felt this girl's pain. She was in deep emotional agony due to the isolation and hurt of being different, of being a young girl and feeling ugly and fat, rejected by her peers. She was in so much pain she was willing to take her own life—or at least to make the statement that she wanted to die.

As I stood watching Patient Y being wheeled away, I suddenly realized that she was, in fact, not alone. There were many others in her age group who were overweight or obese. I wondered how many of these kids were also feeling tremendous psychological pain. How many of them were like Patient Y, depressed and discouraged, hating themselves and their lives, feeling desperate enough to kill themselves rather than suffer any longer?

Where was the hope, I wondered? Why didn't Patient Y just go on a diet and lose some weight? Why kill herself?

There had to be a way to help kids like Patient Y to lose weight, learn to love themselves, and have a decent chance at life. At the time, I became more determined than ever to do something about this dangerous and disabling disease: obesity, and I vowed I would attempt to help overweight kids as well as adults.

Fat Kids

It's a frightening statistic: kids who are overweight are not expected to enjoy the same life span as their parents. In fact, if we don't hurry up and do something about today's generation of overweight children, our kids will not live as long as we do. This will be a historical first, the first generation in North American history to live a shorter life span than the generation before it. And the problem of obesity in youth is becoming global as developed nations see their children growing fatter and less healthy.

Yet, the cause is simple, obvious: young folks are getting fatter because of how and what they are eating.

What *are* they eating? All the Wrong Foods and very few Smart Foods. At home in front of the television or computer, our kids are consuming microwaved convenience foods in trays and over-processed snack foods out of plastic bags. They are drinking large servings of soft drinks with so much sugar or high fructose corn sweeteners that their bodies are becoming hyperactive and insulin resistant. On the go at school or in after-school programs and classes, our kids are grabbing fast foods and junk foods, eating mindlessly and unhealthily. They've grown up with Ronald McDonald, Tony the Tiger, and the Pepsi challenge. They've grown fat eating Happy Meals, donuts in cereal, and supersized snack foods.

It is a sad truth that the modern kid's diet is full of additives and pesticides, artificial colors and flavors, all the Wrong ingredients and few of the Smart ones. And the modern kid does not exercise much, if at all, finding few opportunities between school and sedentary at-home behaviors—like video games, computer games, and TV watching—for outdoor activities that involve running around.

As kids, we had experiences different than those of our children. When we were young, our generation spent a lot of time in the streets or sand lots, backyards and neighborhood parks, playing sports, hide and seek, and a variety of physically demanding games. Our kids—for safety reasons and because their activities must be supervised—are usually at a school desk or on a couch unless they are between the two in the back seat of a SUV. Teenagers are on their cellphones, in class or their cars, rarely out and about on their own two feet in the fresh air, exercising.

The contemporary sedentary and fast food lifestyle does not have to be a given for your children. You can help your kids to *establish healthy eating and exercise behaviors right now*, behaviors that will allow your kids to live long, healthy, fit lives.

The lifestyle changes your family makes to improve everyone's overall health can be fun for you and your kids. That's what my program ThinAdventure is all about: being fit and having fun.

How to Begin the ThinAdventure

Like you or any adult embarking on a weight loss program, your kids should obtain permission from the family doctor before they embark on the ThinAdventure. There is certainly nothing unsafe about eating healthfully and exercising regularly, but it is always a good idea to have your child visit his or her doctor for a physical. Tell your pediatrician about Smart for Life ThinAdventure Healthy Weight Program for kids. Your child's physician may already know about the program and, once he or she understands it, will undoubtedly endorse it heartily.

Next, help your child to select a healthy weight goal. Remember, kids are still sprouting and thus need more food energy for cell development and physical growth. Kids also tend to lose weight more quickly than adults. Their metabolisms tend to be faster and, in most cases, not as inefficient as those of overweight adults. Eating Smart with ThinAdventure will make sure that your kid's metabolism is efficient and appropriate for his or her size and age.

It is exceedingly unwise to select an unrealistic weight goal for your child. Trying to "get skinny" can easily lead to years of unhealthy behaviors associated with food and body image. Eating disorders like bulimia and anorexia often begin with restrictive diets and unrealistic weight goals. Too many kids ruin their lives and their health with these prevalent food and body obsessions, both girls and, increasingly, boys.

Don't let this happen to your kid. Keep the emphasis on healthy eating, exercising, and a fit body. When overweight children come to see me at a Smart for Life Weight Management Center, I do not set a goal weight. Help your child change activity and eating behaviors, without making him or her feel deprived or obsessed about food.

You can use the BMI Tables to help your kid calculate his or her BMI.

BMI Calculation: Table, Boys & Girls

To calculate your BMI, follow these simple directons: 1. Find your height in the left hand column 2. Find your approximate weight 3. Use a finger to follow across and up to your BMI number 4. Use the charts to the right (separate for boys and girls) to find where you fall by age and BMI number. 5. If you are "Very Overweight" or "Overweight", there is work to be done. Start by following the THINADVENTURE™ plan to lose the weight.

Example for a 12 yr old girl:	Height: 4'9" tall Weight: 106 pounds	BMI: 23

BMI ▶ / Weight (pounds)	13	14	15	16	17	18	19	20	21	22	23	24	25	26	27	28	29	30	31	32	33	34	35	36
33" (2'9")	20	21	23	24	26	27	29	30	32	34	35	37	38	40	41	43	44	46	48	49	51	52	54	55
34" (2'10")	21	23	24	26	27	29	31	32	34	36	37	39	41	42	44	46	47	49	50	52	54	55	57	59
35" (2'11")	22	24	26	27	29	31	33	34	36	38	40	41	43	45	47	48	50	52	54	55	57	59	60	62
36" (3'0")	23	25	27	29	31	33	35	36	38	40	42	44	46	47	49	51	53	55	57	58	60	62	64	66
37" (3'1")	25	27	29	31	33	35	37	38	40	42	44	46	48	50	52	54	56	58	60	62	64	66	68	70
38" (3'2")	26	28	30	32	34	36	39	41	43	45	47	49	51	53	55	57	59	61	63	65	67	69	71	73
39" (3'3")	28	30	32	34	36	38	41	43	45	47	49	51	54	56	58	60	62	64	67	69	71	73	75	77
40" (3'4")	29	31	34	36	38	40	43	45	47	50	52	54	56	59	61	63	66	68	70	72	75	77	79	81
41" (3'5")	31	33	35	38	40	43	45	47	50	52	54	57	59	62	64	66	69	71	74	76	78	81	83	86
42" (3'6")	32	35	37	40	42	45	47	50	52	55	57	60	62	65	67	70	72	75	77	80	82	85	87	90
43" (3'7")	34	36	39	42	44	47	49	52	55	57	60	63	65	68	71	73	76	78	81	84	86	89	92	94
44" (3'8")	35	38	41	44	46	49	52	55	57	60	63	66	68	71	74	77	79	82	85	88	90	93	96	99
45" (3'9")	37	40	43	46	48	51	54	57	60	63	66	69	72	74	77	80	83	86	89	92	95	97	100	103
46" (3'10")	39	42	45	48	51	54	57	60	63	66	69	72	75	78	81	84	87	90	93	96	99	102	105	108
47" (3'11")	40	43	47	50	53	56	59	62	65	69	72	75	78	81	84	87	91	94	97	100	103	106	109	113
48" (4'0")	42	45	49	52	55	58	62	65	68	72	75	78	81	85	88	91	95	98	101	104	108	111	114	117
49" (4'1")	44	47	51	54	58	61	64	68	71	75	78	81	85	88	92	95	99	102	105	109	112	116	119	122
50" (4'2")	46	49	53	56	60	64	67	71	74	78	81	85	88	92	96	99	103	106	110	113	117	120	124	128
51" (4'3")	48	51	55	59	62	66	70	73	77	81	85	88	92	96	99	103	107	110	114	118	122	125	129	133
52" (4'4")	50	53	57	61	65	69	73	76	80	84	88	92	96	100	103	107	111	115	119	123	126	130	134	138
53" (4'5")	51	55	59	63	67	71	75	79	83	87	91	95	99	103	107	111	115	119	123	127	131	135	139	143
54" (4'6")	53	58	62	66	70	74	78	82	87	91	95	99	103	107	111	116	120	124	128	132	136	141	145	149
55" (4'7")	55	60	64	68	73	77	81	86	90	94	98	103	107	111	116	120	124	129	133	137	141	146	150	154
56" (4'8")	57	62	66	71	75	80	84	89	93	98	102	107	111	115	120	124	129	133	138	142	147	151	156	160
57' (4'9")	60	64	69	73	78	83	87	92	97	101	106	110	115	120	124	129	134	138	143	147	152	157	161	166
58' (4'10")	62	66	71	76	81	86	90	95	100	105	110	114	119	124	129	133	138	143	148	153	157	162	167	172
59' (4'11")	64	69	74	79	84	89	94	99	103	108	113	118	123	128	133	138	143	148	153	158	163	168	173	178
60" (5'0")	66	71	76	81	87	92	97	102	107	112	117	122	128	133	138	143	148	153	158	163	168	174	179	184
61" (5'1")	68	74	79	84	89	95	100	105	111	116	121	127	132	137	142	148	153	158	164	169	174	179	185	190
62" (5'2")	71	76	82	87	92	98	103	109	114	120	125	131	136	142	147	153	158	164	169	174	180	185	191	196
63" (5'3")	73	79	84	90	95	101	107	112	118	124	129	135	141	146	152	158	163	169	175	180	186	191	197	203
64" (5'4")	75	81	87	93	99	104	110	116	122	128	134	139	145	151	157	163	168	174	180	186	192	198	203	209
65' (5'5")	78	84	90	96	102	108	114	120	126	132	138	144	150	156	162	168	174	180	186	192	198	204	210	216
66' (5'6")	80	86	92	99	105	111	117	123	130	136	142	148	154	161	167	173	179	185	192	198	204	210	216	223
67' (5'7")	83	89	95	102	108	114	121	127	134	140	146	153	159	166	172	178	185	191	197	204	210	217	223	229
68' (5'8")	85	92	98	105	111	118	124	131	138	144	151	157	164	171	177	184	190	197	203	210	217	223	230	236
69' (5'9")	88	94	101	108	115	121	128	135	142	148	155	162	169	176	182	189	196	203	209	216	223	230	237	243
70' (5'10")	90	97	104	111	118	125	132	139	146	153	160	167	174	181	188	195	202	209	216	223	230	236	243	250
71' (5'11")	93	100	107	114	121	129	136	143	150	157	164	172	179	186	193	200	207	215	222	229	236	243	250	258
72' (6'0")	95	103	110	117	125	132	140	147	154	162	169	176	184	191	199	206	213	221	228	235	243	250	258	265

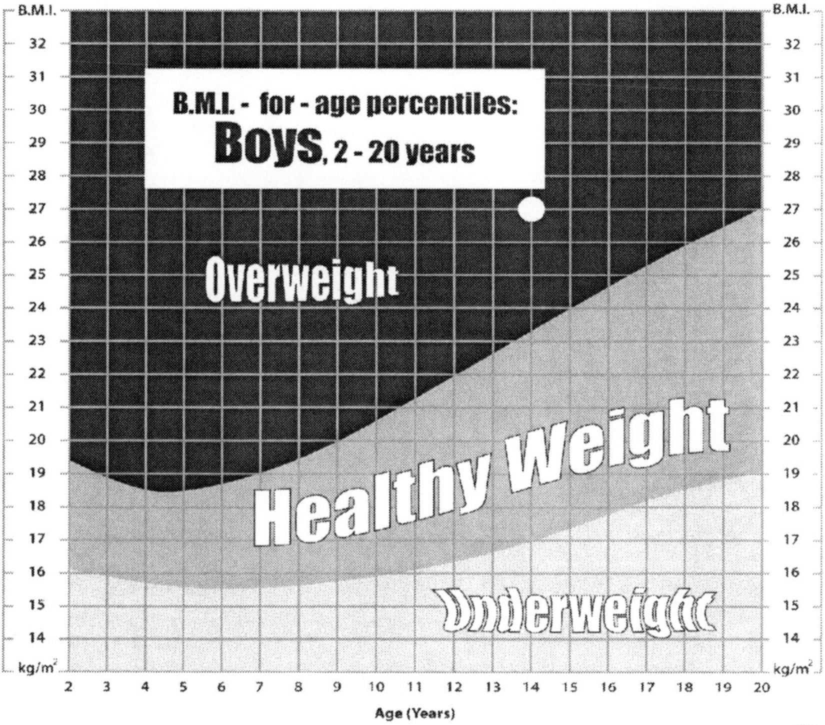

Once you have your BMI number follow these easy directions:

1. Find your age at the bottom of the chart.
2. Find your BMI on the right column of the chart.
3. Use 2 fingers to follow across and down to see where you fall.

Example:
BMI: 27
Age: 14
Very Overweight

Published May 20, 2000 (modified 10/16/00)
SOURCE: Designed by the National Center for Health Statistics in collaboration with the National Center for Chronic Disease Prevention and Health Promotion (2000)

With kids, the best plan is to allow for growth and shoot for the healthy weight range for your child's age and height, but let them focus on their own behaviors rather than on the scale. Kids will lose weight, stop losing weight, grow taller, and slim down. There is no need to obsess over the numbers on the scale. Weight loss in kids often occurs in spurts, and you don't want your child to feel discouraged. Kids may plateau as they grow, not losing weight but gaining inches, muscle, and bone. This can mask fat loss.

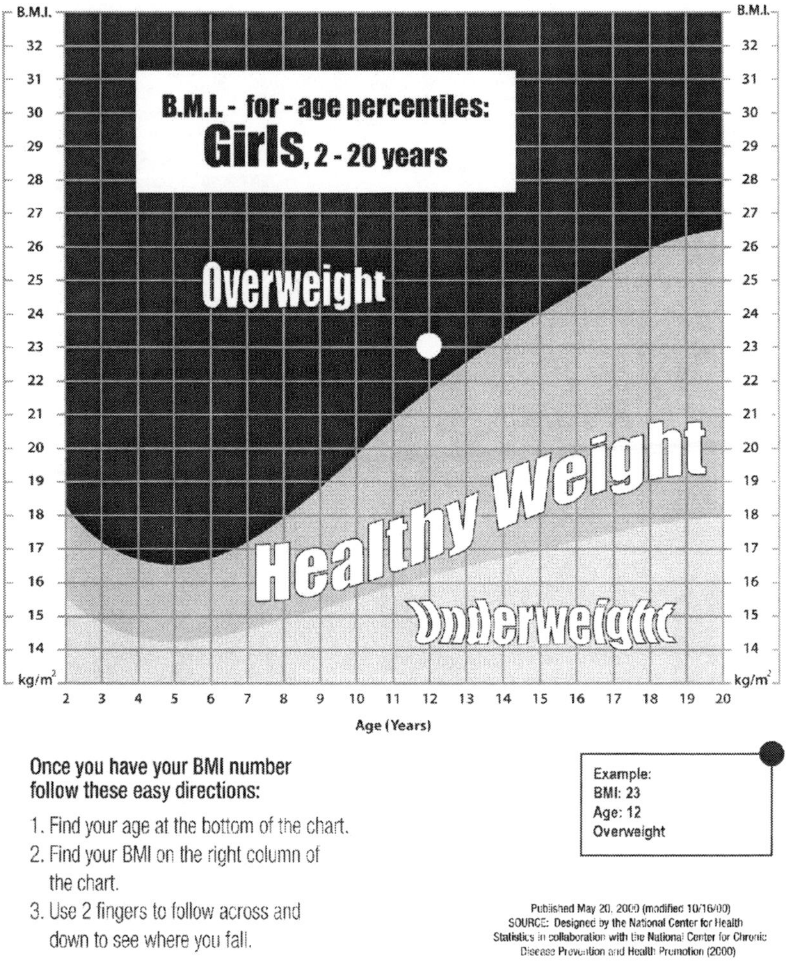

Instead, judge the physical changes that are occurring by having your child note how clothes fit. Ask your child to take notice of how he or she feels. How energetic is your son or daughter? How are school behavior and socializing? These are better markers for success for kids on weight loss programs.

Let me warn you: your kids will eat Wrong Foods sometimes. This is normal behavior. My advice to you is to ignore the occasional cheat and encourage your child to eat healthy and feel good about him or herself. Focusing on errors will provide negative reinforcement. Kids who are trying to slim down need positive reinforcement. It's your job as parent to provide as much enthusiasm, support, and positive feedback as you can give.

ThinAdventure for the Family

The ThinAdventure program is a child's version of Smart for Life. The program is designed to provide the right amounts of healthful protein, carbohydrate, and fat for kids and teens. ThinAdventure allows for proper hunger control, steady weight loss, and adequate nutrition. Make sure your child follows the program exactly to see the best results.

Some of the basics are identical to the adult program:

*eat six small meals and snacks throughout the day plus a healthy dinner at night

*drink plenty of water (6 to 8 eight-ounce glasses a day)

*eat natural foods that do not have additives, preservatives, or artificial ingredients

*eat slowly and do not overeat, eating only when hungry and stopping before feeling full

Just like you, your child needs to learn how to control his or her appetite, eat moderately when hungry, and to make healthy food choices. You already know these basics from reading the previous chapters, so you can explain them to your child.

However, keep in mind there are differences in the program for children: more fruit is included; protein serving sizes vary depending on the child's age; snacks can include all-natural popcorn that you or your child prepare in the microwave; and snacks may be eaten after dinner and before bed. Growing kids need food before bed while adults do not. Also, overweight kids who are losing weight do need to exercise.

If your child is not enrolled in a sports program, you might want to find something suitable for your child to do outside or in a gym. Make sure the activity is one your child enjoys. Do not force your kid to play sports he or she hates. Such regimentation will backfire and make life miserable for all concerned.

As their bodies change, kids' interests adjust in surprising ways. As he or she loses weight, sports may become an increasingly attractive way to spend time.

In the meantime, consider the following activities and discuss with your kid:

*bike riding

*skateboarding

*roller-skating

*swimming

*yoga classes

*dance classes

*jump-rope and small weights for an at-home gym

*swings and playground activities

*walking to and from school, if safe

*mall walking

*lawn mowing and gardening

*exercise while watching TV

The amount of food energy your child needs daily depends on his or her age and activity level. Use the following chart to plan your child's meals and snacks. Note that the snacks should be eaten one at a time, spaced throughout the day. If you kid plays sports, be sure to include a snack beforehand. If the sports program is strenuous, your child can add an additional snack to the menu.

Table A (Follow according to your age) More details on following pages.

5-8 YEARS OLD (MINIMUM OF 6-8 CUPS OF WATER A DAY)

Breakfast	Lunch	Dinner	Snacks (1 at a time; spaced throughout the day)
1 Fruit	1 Smart Cookie	4 oz. Protein	1 Fruit
1 Smart Cookie or	or the equivalent	2 vegetables	2 cups of Low-fat Popcorn
the equivalent	1 Sm. Salad	1 Fruit	1 Smart Cookie or equivalent (eaten any time)
			1 cup of Skim Milk

8-10 YEARS OLD (MINIMUM OF 6-8 CUPS OF WATER A DAY)

Breakfast	Lunch	Dinner	Snacks (1 at a time; spaced throughout the day)
1 Fruit	2 Smart Cookies or	5 oz. Protein	1 Fruit
1 Smart Cookie or	the equivalent	2 vegetables	2 cups of Low-fat Popcorn
the equivalent	1 Sm. Salad	1 Fruit	1 Smart Cookie or equivalent (eaten any time)
			1 cup of Skim Milk

10-12 YEARS OLD (MINIMUM OF 8 CUPS OF WATER A DAY)

Breakfast	Lunch	Dinner	Snacks (1 at a time; spaced throughout the day)
1 Fruit	2 Smart Cookies or	6-8 oz. Protein	1 Fruit
2 Smart Cookies or	the equivalent	2 vegetables	2 cups of Low-fat Popcorn
the equivalent	1 Sm. Salad	1 Fruit	2 Smart Cookies or equivalent (eaten any time)
			1 cup of Skim Milk

12-14 YEARS OLD (MINIMUM OF 8 CUPS OF WATER A DAY)

Breakfast	Lunch	Dinner	Snacks (1 at a time; spaced throughout the day)
1 Fruit	2-4 oz. Protein	6-8 oz. Protein	1 Fruit
2 Smart Cookies or	2 Smart Cookies or	2 vegetables	2 cups of Low-fat Popcorn
the equivalent	the equivalent	1 Fruit	2 Smart Cookies or equivalent (eaten any time)
	1 Sm. Salad		1 cup of Skim Milk

Unlimited green vegetables may be eaten any time of day at least 5 servings or more per day (see more information about serving sizes in the vegetable category).

If you are on the Smart for Life program, you will be serving your child the Smart Foods you are eating and NOT serving them the Wrong Foods you, too, are avoiding. Because you have already destocked your pantry, the change in family meals and snacks should not be too dramatic. Refer to the Smart Foods, Wrong Foods, and Superfoods lists provided in Chapter 3 to give you and your child the guidance required. If you haven't already done so, post these lists on your refrigerator or kitchen cabinet.

When shopping, select a wide variety of natural and unsweetened fruit for your kids: apples and applesauce, peaches, pears, berries, papaya, mango, dried fruits like organic dates and raisins, fresh pomegranate slices, pineapple chunks, melon, and citrus. Be sure your child consumes one and one-half cups of fruit daily. All children benefit from the nutrients found in fresh fruit.

I recommend you give your child a daily vitamin and mineral supplement. This will provide nutrition insurance while he or she is on the ThinAdventure. Most parents continue to provide nutrition supplementation after weight has been lost. When meals or snacks are missed or if vegetables are not eaten in adequate amounts (all too common for kids), nutrition supplements can prove helpful.

ThinAdventure Food Tips: Fruit

Here are the fruit servings I recommend for my young patients with a daily total of one and one-half cups:

*1/2 medium size fruit such as orange, grapefruit, apple, pear, banana

*1/2 cup sliced banana

*1/2 cup unsweetened fruit cocktail, grapes, applesauce

*1/2 cup unsweetened berries or cherries

*1/2 cup sliced or diced orange, tangerine, melon, mango

*1/2 cup sliced or diced peach, pear, pineapple, plum, kiwi

*1/2 cup dried fruits like raisins, dates, figs

*1/2 cup unsweetened fruit juice

*fruit smoothie with fresh fruit and fruit juice (total 1/2 cup)

Variety is key. Let your kids try new fruits like kiwi, mango, and pomegranate. Read labels carefully to avoid sweetened fruit and sweetened fruit juices.

ThinAdventure Food Tips: Snacks

My young patients usually eat their snacks as follows: one snack in the afternoon, one after dinner, and one when needed during the day or evening. Some kids get hungry before bed; others like to eat something right after school. How your child divides up his or her snacks will be determined on an individual basis.

Some kids love milk. If your child prefers milk to fruit, you can allow him or her to drink an 8-ounce glass of fat-free milk as a snack instead of fruit. Low-fat soy milk is also acceptable. Low-fat unsweetened yogurt can work as a snack as well. Kids need at least one serving of dairy food or soy milk daily to meet their nutrient needs.

Kids like nuts, and these make an excellent snack choice. You can prepare small Ziploc bags of walnuts, almonds, or cashews to send with your kids to school or sports. If they will eat them, raw veggie sticks also make an excellent snack, especially if served with low-fat cheese, low-fat cottage cheese, or low-fat sour cream. Homemade hummus makes a great dip. Some kids love the taste of almond milk. Buy a carton and see if your kids like the taste.

ThinAdventure Food Tips: Breakfasts

High protein breakfasts are essential to proper brain function, and protein is especially important for kids. But most kids eat sugary cereals, donuts, pastries, and toaster pastries instead, Wrong Foods that boost blood sugar and over-stimulate insulin response. Eating nutrient poor breakfasts is a terrible habit for your kids to have—it's unhealthy at any age. It is essential for you to reform your kids' breakfast habits now and for life.

Studies show kids who eat sound breakfasts do better in school. You should notice a significant difference in your child's attention span and behavior once you eliminate high sugar cereals and over-sweetened foodstuffs from the breakfast table. Some kids diagnosed with attention deficit disorders like ADD and ADHD are actually high on food additives and sweeteners. Once such unhealthy ingredients are removed from their diets, kids usually begin to behave in more normal parameters.

Read the following story about one of my young patients, a striking example of how breakfast can influence a child's overall health.

Jacey and ADD

When Jacey's mother came to see me at the Smart for Life Weight Management Center in Boca Raton, she brought her 10-year-old daughter with her. Jacey's mother was seriously overweight and needed to lose a significant amount of weight. Her child was fat, too, but I did not say anything about the child. When I first meet a patient, we focus on him or her. After a week or two, we talk about the rest of the family.

However, Jacey's mom surprised me during that first consultation by pointing to her daughter and asking me without hesitation, "Is there anything you can do for my child? Can you help her lose weight, too?"

"Sure," I responded. I was happy to help.

Parents need to be aware of their kids' weight issues and seek help if they are unable to assist their children to attain and maintain a healthy weight. Many times, the family physician will not point out the need for young patients to lose weight. To me, that is like a patient coming to a doctor with a sprained ankle and a neck fracture and having the physician tend to the ankle while ignoring the neck. This is what I see happening in modern medicine today, and I think such willful avoidance is inexcusable. Doctors need to speak up and inform their patients how dangerous it is for kids to be overweight.

When I worked as an emergency room doctor, we would often see overweight or obese children for minor ailments like rashes and viruses. We might give the parent a cream for the rash, or we would discuss the illness and advise the parent on proper care. However, *whenever a child came in who was overweight, the main issue was the obesity.* Everyone in the ER could see the main problem and knew the dangers the condition posed to the child. Yet, nobody would say anything to the parents. No physician in the ER would say to the mother, "Look: your child is overweight. Here is the cream for the rash. That rash will disappear. But you need to do something about your child's obesity. Don't ignore the problem. Her weight is a major issue that can impact your child's entire future."

I learned through experience that it is the doctor's responsibility to bring the child's welfare to the attention of the parents, so I am not shy about telling parents to take notice and do something if their kid is overweight.

In Jacey's case, her mother was aware of the problem and asking for my help, so I gave her a handbook for our ThinAdventure weight program for kids, which included much of the information in this chapter. I explained the ThinAdventure Healthy Weight program to Jacey's mom and showed her the healthy products available for Jacey to eat. I usually consult at no cost to my patients who want to help their kids lose weight. ThinAdventure is free, and the products we make for kids on the program are available at affordable prices.

The next week, Jacey and her mom returned to the Smart for Life Weight Management Center. Jacey's mom had lost 7 pounds, and she was thrilled. But Jacey had not lost any weight. I asked the girl if she was following the program, and she said yes, she was. I told the mother that this sometimes happens, and we should give the program another week before looking for physical causes.

When they returned the next week, however, neither had lost

any weight. In fact, Jacey had gained a pound. They both insisted they were following the program, and I doubted that they were lying. The problem was not metabolic because the mother had lost 7 pounds the week before. I knew there had to be a dietary error they were making, one they were making together while not understanding the impact on their weight. There was something they were both doing that was sabotaging their progress, something simple but invisible to the mother and the daughter.

At this point, I became a detective and asked Jacey's mother some questions. "What did you have for dinner last night?" I asked her, and she told me. The dinner had been excellent, a perfect choice for someone on the Smart for Life weight loss program.

"Okay, so what did you two have for lunch?" I asked her. Their lunches were equally appropriate. Both of them had been following the program perfectly.

And then I struck pay dirt: "What did you have for breakfast?" I asked.

"Oh," answered Jacey's mother, "we drive to the local cafe every morning and have a *frappucino venti.* We each have one," she told me.

Aha! A frappucino is an iced coffee drink made with milk, sugar, and coffee. The *venti* is 20 to 24 ounces of this potent mixture and may contain 5 grams of fat and 160 milligrams of caffeine. It packs a caloric wallop, too, with around 450 calories per very tall drink, but many people think that a coffee drink like this is simply "coffee," which is non-caloric and non-fattening. Wrong!

I explained the facts to Jacey and her mother, and we looked together at the caloric and fat contents of their daily breakfast drink on the coffee chain company's website. When I told Jacey's mom she was overdosing herself and her child with caffeine, a nervous system stimulant, she was shocked. And then she told me something quite interesting.

"Jacey is on medication for Attention Deficit Disorder."

No surprise. The excessive intakes of sugar and caffeine had to be contributing to if not causing the child's neurological issues. For a 10-year-old child, consuming such strong coffee drinks on a daily basis provides a significant overload for the developing nervous system. There was little doubt in my mind Jacey's ADD would diminish or disappear entirely once she cut the coffee milkshakes and began to eat a healthy diet.

We discussed healthy breakfast options including fruit and high protein cereals.

The next time Jacey and her mom came to see me, they both looked thinner and healthier. Sure enough, the mother had lost several pounds. And Jacey was down 4 pounds! There had been some noticeable improvements in Jacey's behavior in school and at home, the mother informed me. And frappucino was no longer on the menu.

After a month on the program, Jacey's mother took her to the family physician and asked if they might wean her off the ADD medication. This was accomplished, and Jacey felt fine. Her behavioral and learning problems had disappeared.

Now I know enough to ask some specific questions when my patients bring in overweight children, and it has become part of my mission to educate parents about keeping their kids in good shape. Sometimes all a kid needs is a change in eating habits to improve overall health. Help your kid to eat a healthier diet and you might be surprised to find the ADD medication may no longer be on the menu, either.

Smart breakfasts might include high-protein cereals like kashi or ThinAdventure cereal with a serving of fruit or an egg white omelet with diced veggies. Use the recipes in Chapter 6 to create healthy morning meals for your kids.

ThinAdventure Food Tips: Lunches and Dinners

Sandwiches are off the menu, and healthy foods are on the menu. Skip the pizza, burgers, and fries in favor of veggies and protein like lean chicken or tuna. Get your kids hooked on chef's salads made with low-fat cheese and olive oil dressing. Introduce your kids to oven-baked zucchini slices and fruit-yogurt smoothies. Vary the menu, and they will enjoy their new non-sandwich, non-fast food fare.

Dinner will be a lot like yours with the protein amount dependent on your child's age. However, the menu will consist of lean protein (chicken, fish, seafood, etc.) plus vegetables. Raw salads and unlimited vegetables can be eaten throughout the day as much as desired. In total, your kid should have a minimum of five cups of vegetables every day.

Vegetables can be the most difficult aspect of the ThinAdventure program. Kids don't usually eat this much produce, and some kids just don't like veggies. Remember, your child will not change his or her habits overnight, but with patience and persistence, he or she will begin to eat more healthfully. Set a good example, make the veggies as attractive as possible, and serve them at lunch and dinner. If your child is hungry, he or she will begin to eat these foods. And, if they are anything like my kids, they will learn to love their veggies.

Use the following charts to determine the allotted amounts of vegetables your child may eat each day.

Unlimited Vegetables—eat freely:

arugula

bok choy

Brussels sprouts

cabbage

cauliflower

celery

chives

cucumber

endive

greens—collards, mustard, turnip

kale

lettuce

mushrooms

peppers-green

purslane

radicchio

radishes

spinach

sprouts

Swiss chard

watercress

zucchini

Limited Vegetables—1/2 cup per serving:

asparagus

beets

broccoli

carrots (2 large)

chickpeas

corn

edamame

eggplant

garlic (1 clove)

green beans

leeks

legumes—black beans, soy beans, kidney beans, navy beans, lentils, split peas

okra

onions

peas

peapods, snow peas

peppers—red and yellow

pickles (1 spear)

scallions

sea vegetables and seaweed

squash

tomato (1 large)

Veggies may be eaten raw, steamed, boiled, or baked without butter. Include veggies in shakes and soups. Substitute salads for a serving of vegetables as often as your child would like. Dress with olive oil, balsamic vinegar, sea salt, and black pepper. My kids love salads and veggies prepared this way.

Do not give your children beef, pork, veal, or lamb. No egg yolk either. These foods are high in saturated fats and cholesterol and do not provide any nutrients your kids can't get from lower fat foods. Be sure to bake, broil, or grill lean cuts of chicken or turkey without skin. You can buy natural deli chicken and turkey without additives at the health food store. Bake, broil, or grill fish and seafood without butter or rich sauces. On occasion, treat your kids to lean buffalo or ostrich meat. The kids may squeal, but your family will enjoy the delicious flavor of wild meat. It's natural and naturally good for you if eaten only once in a while.

Limit your child's intake of canned tuna and other high-mercury fish to once a week or less. These fish are lower in mercury content: anchovies, conch, herring, Atlantic mackerel, salmon, Atlantic sardines, sturgeon, fresh blue fin tuna, and lean white fish like flounder and sole or shellfish like shrimp, scallops, crab, clams, etc.

Serve legumes in salads, soups, and stews. Introduce hummus. Your kids will love it. See if your kids will eat miso. It's good for digestion and immune function. Serve them tofu or tempeh, soft soybean curd that makes a delicious protein addition to veggies and casseroles. Check out the recipes in Chapter 6.

Add low-fat cheeses to veggie dishes for a protein boost. Most kids love cheese even when the fat has been removed. At your local supermarket, you can find Kraft fat-free cheeses (American and sharp cheddar, shredded and slices), Polly-O fat-free mozzarella, and Borden's sliced fat-free cheeses (American, Swiss, and cheddar). Read labels and make sure the cheese you buy contains 0% fat, 2 grams of carbohydrate, and 5 grams of protein.

ThinAdventure Exercise Tips

Calisthenics used to be a part of every kids' gym class at school. Budget cuts and overcrowded classes have reduced the amount of physical activity offered during the school day in most educational settings. The loss of exercise in school is a shame and a contributing factor to the increase in childhood obesity.

But you can help your kid at home. See if you can interest your child in doing some easy, fun calisthenics. You might tell your child he or she can practice jumping jacks, toe-touches, sit-ups, and push-ups whenever boring commercials are on TV. Better yet, exercise with your child each day instead of parking him or her in front of the television.

Losing excess weight can change your child's life. A healthy weight can result in significant improvements in self-esteem, social life, college choices, and job opportunities. Being thinner can mean the difference between a lifetime of illness and chronic disease and one of health and success. Weight loss *now* can mean your kid could live to be 100 or more. We have made the advances in medicine and technology necessary to provide the next generation with expanded life spans. Your kid could join the centurions, a generation of the super-fit who will lead us into the future.

Obviously, helping your child to get fit and stay fit is one of the most important tasks you can do as a parent. When your child feels better about life, you will, too.

My patient Allie Z. and her proud dad illustrate the truth of this perfectly.

Allie Z.

Joe Z. is a well-known radio disc jockey with a large fan base. He's a nice guy, and I enjoyed helping him with his weight problem. He had around 70 pounds to lose and found Smart for Life to be a good fit for his hectic schedule. He liked the products and thought the program was easy to follow.

After a few months on the program, Joe had lost 45 pounds, and he felt great. He was happier around the house, and his family noticed.

Then his 14 year old daughter Allie asked if she could try the program, too.

When Allie first came to see me at the Smart for Life Weight Management Center in Boca Raton, Florida, she was shy and awkward. She was a good student, but, she told me in her quiet voice, she was unhappy in school. She had always been one of those children the other kids teased and made fun of because of her weight.

Allie was self-conscious about her appearance and was ashamed to admit she had a weight problem. But once she decided to do something about it with Smart for Life, there was no stopping her. And after losing 6 pounds during her first week on the program, Allie was hooked.

In only 10 weeks, this determined young woman lost almost 30 pounds.

I immediately noticed a significant change in her personality. Allie began to smile a lot. She was no longer awkward, and she engaged me and my staff, opening up to us and sharing her thoughts. "The ThinAdventure program is so easy to follow," she told us. "I love the carrot cupcakes and the ThinAdventure shakes. And I'm not hungry like I used to be at school or on the weekends."

Her father was thrilled. He remained on the program, too, and eventually lost the entire 70 pounds he wanted to shed. But he was more excited about his daughter's success. He told me how she had changed into a happier, more vibrant person. Joe had been so sad when his lovely girl was overweight, lonely, and unhappy. Now the whole family felt better.

Allie didn't require any support from us, probably because she had all the encouragement she needed at home. She would come into the Smart for Life Weight Management Center, weigh in, pick up her ThinAdventure products, and chat about her life. "I feel a lot better about myself when I go places like school, and this seems to be only the beginning!" she told me one day.

Allie Z. did not need medication or counseling. She just needed to learn how to eat healthy foods in the right amounts. At Smart for Life, we see this often with children who are overweight. They don't need stern lectures, strict regimens, or a focus on cutting calories. Once kids start eating Smart on a diet of healthy foods, they feel better and look better. And they lose weight.

Everybody wins.

Appendix A: Recommended Reading

The following books can enhance your knowledge of the science behind the Smart for Life program. You might want to read these books for more information on topics such as metabolic dysfunction and food messaging, the glycemic index for foods, fructose and weight gain, gut microflora and health, green eating as healthy eating, food industry politics, food and the environment, and other important food issues.

Gary Taubes. *Why We Get Fat.* Knopf, 2011.

Leo Galland. *The Fat Resistance Diet.* Broadway, 2005.

Ron Rosedale. *The Rosedale Diet.* Harper Resource, 2004.

William Bennett and Joel Gurin. *The Dieter's Dilemma: Eating Less and Weighing More.* Basic Books, 1982.

Jeffrey Bland. *Genetic Nutritioneering.* McGraw Hill, 1999.

Rick Gallop. *The Glycemic Index Diet.* Virgin Books, 2007.

Steven Gundry. *Dr. Gundry's Diet Evolution.* Crown, 2008.

Bradley Willcox, D. Craig Willcox, and Makoto Suzuki. *The Okinawa Diet Plan.* Clarkson Potter, 2004.

Greg Critzer. *Fat Land.* Mariner, 2003.

David Kessler. *The End of Over-eating.* Rodale, 2009.

Michael D. Gershon. *The Second Brain.* Harper, 1999.

Michael Pollan. *The Omnivore's Dilemma.* Penguin, 2006.

Steve Ettlinger. *Twinkie, Deconstructed.* Plume, 2007.

Marion Nestle. *Food Politics.* University of California Press, 2001.

Eric Schlosser. *Fast Food Nation.* Harper Perennial, 2004.

Michele Simon. *Appetite for Profit: How the Food Industry Undermines our Health.* Nation Books, 2006.

Hank Cardello. *Stuffed: An Insider's Look at Who's (Really) Making America Fat.* Ecco, 2009.

The following references from scientific journals include studies on the influence of physical activity on body weight:

Fogelholm, M. and K. Kukkonen-Harjula. 2000. "Does physical activity prevent weight gain—A systemic review." *Obesity Reviews.* Oct;1(2):95-111.

Segal, K.R. and F.X. Pi-Sunyer. 1989. "Exercise and obesity," *Medical Clinics of North America,* Jan;73 (1):217-36.

Williams, P.T. and P.D. Wood. 2006. "The effects of changing exercise levels on weight and age-related weight gain." *International Journal of Obesity.* Mar;30(3):543-51.

The references below include some very interesting studies on appetite regulation, nutrition and weight loss, diet and disease, and related topics of interest.

Kuate, D. et al. 2010. "The use of LeptiCore in reducing fat gain and managing weight loss in patients with metabolic syndrome." *Lipids in Health and Disease.* Feb;19(9):20.

Farooqi, I.S. and S. O'Rahilly. 2009. "Leptin: A pivotal regulator of human energy homeostasis." *American Journal of Clinical Nutrition.* Mar;89(3):980S-984S.

Berthoud. H. 2005. "A new role for leptin as a direct satiety signal from the stomach." *American Journal of Physiology—Regulatory, Integrative and Comparative Physiology.* Apr;288(4):R796-R797.

Keim, N.L. et al. 1998. "Relation between circulating leptin concentrations and appetite during a prolonged, moderate energy deficit in women." *American Journal of Clinical Nutrition.* Oct;68(4):794-801.

Garrow, J.S. et al. 1981. "The effect of meal frequency and protein concentration on the composition of the weight lost by obese subjects." *British Journal of Nutrition.* 45(1): 5-15.

Jenkins, D.A. et al. 2008. "Effect of a low-glycemic index or a high-cereal fiber diet on type 2 diabetes." *Journal of the American Medical Association.* Dec 17; 300(23):2742-2753.

Kiecolt-Glaser, J.K. et al. 2007. "Depressive symptoms, omega 6:omega 3 fatty acids, and inflammation in older adults." *Psychosomatic Medicine.* 69(3):217-224.

Van der Tempel, H. et al. 1990. "Effects of fish oil supplementation in rheumatoid arthritis," *Annals of Rheumatic Diseases.* 49(2):76-80.

Hill, A.M. et al. 2007. "Combining fish-oil supplements with regular aerobic exercise improves body composition and cardiovascular disease risk factors."

American Journal of Clinical Nutrition. May;85(5):1267-1274.

Barber, N. 2010. "Top reasons Americans are food obsessed." *Psychology Today.*

The Human Beast blog, September 16, 2010.

Corsica, J.A. and M.L. Pelchat. 2010. "Food addiction: True or false?" *Current Opinion in Gastroenterology.* Mar;26(2):165-169.

Johnson, P.M. and P.J. Kenny. 2010. "Dopamine D2 receptors in addiction-like reward dysfunction and compulsive eating in obese rats." *Nature Neuroscience.* Mar(13): 635-641.

Barr, E.L. et al. 2007. "Risk of cardiovascular and all-cause mortality in individuals with diabetes mellitus, impaired fasting glucose and impaired glucose tolerance." *Circulation.* Jul 10;116:151-157.

Anderson, J.W. and E.C. Konz. 2001. "Obesity and disease management: Effects of weight loss on comorbid conditions." *Obesity*

Research. Nov;9(4):326S-334S.

Must, A. et al. 1999. "The disease burden associated with overweight and obesity."

Journal of the American Medical Association. Oct 27;282(16):1523-1529.

Berrino, F. 2002. "Western diet and Alzheimer's disease." *Epidemiologia E Prevenzione.* May-June;26(3):107-115.

Petanceska, S.A. 2007. "Exploring the links between obesity and Alzheimer's disease." *Current Alzheimer Research.* April;4(2):95-134.

Hertz-Picciotto, I. and D. Amaral. 2011. "International Meeting for Autism Research." May 11, presentations.

Masoro, E.J. et al. 1982. "Action of food restriction in delaying the aging process."

Proceedings of the National Academy of Science. Jul 1;79(13):4239-4241.

Ross, M.H. 1972. "Length of life and caloric intake." *American Journal of Clinical Nutrition.* Aug;25(8):834-838.

Schoonover, H. and M. Muller. 2006. "Food without thought: How U.S. farm policy contributes to obesity." Institute for Agriculture and Trade Policy, 1-14.

McMichael, A.J. et al. 2007. "Food, livestock production, energy, climate change, and health." *The Lancet.* Oct 6;370(9594):1253-1263.

Pimentel, D. et al. 2009. "Food versus biofuels: environmental and economic costs." *Human Ecology.* 37(1):1-12.

Lawson, E.A. et al. 2011. "Appetite regulating hormones cortisol and peptide YY are associated with disordered eating psychopathology, independent of body mass index." *European Journal of Endocrinology.* Feb;164(2):253-261.

Schwenke, D. 2010. "Seasonal fluctuations in weight is not associated with weight gain." *Circulation.* 122:A21291.

Hanson, L.A. et al. 1999. "Normal microbial flora of the gut and the immune system" in *Probiotics, Other Nutritional Factors and Intestinal*

Microflora. Nestle Nutrition Workshop series, Volume 42.

Isolauri, E. 2001. "Probiotics: effects on immunity. *American Journal of Clinical Nutrition.* Feb;73(2):444S-450S.

Cani, P.D. et al. 2008. "Role of gut microflora in the development of obesity and insulin resistance following high-fat diet feeding." *Pathologie Biologie* 56:305-309.

National Institute on Aging. 2009. "Restricting caloric intake may improve the body's metabolic efficiency." *Recognition of Excellence in Aging Research Committee Report*, Senate Congressional Report S. Rept. 527-110.

Civitarese, A. et al. 2007. "Calorie restriction increases muscle mitochondrial biogenesis in healthy humans." *Public Library of Science, Medicine.* 4(3):e76.

Heilbronn, L.K. et al. 2006. "Effect of 6-month calorie restriction on biomarkers of longevity, metabolic adaptation, and oxidative stress in overweight individuals." *Journal of the American Medical Association.* Apr 5;295(13):1539-1548.

Ogden, C. and M. Carroll. 2010. "Prevalence of obesity among children and adolescents: United States trends 1963-1965 through 2007-2008." Centers for Disease Control and Prevention, National Health and Nutrition Examination Survey Data.

American Heart Association. 2011. "Overweight children." www.heart.org

Your Smart for Life Weight Tracker
Fill in your progress.

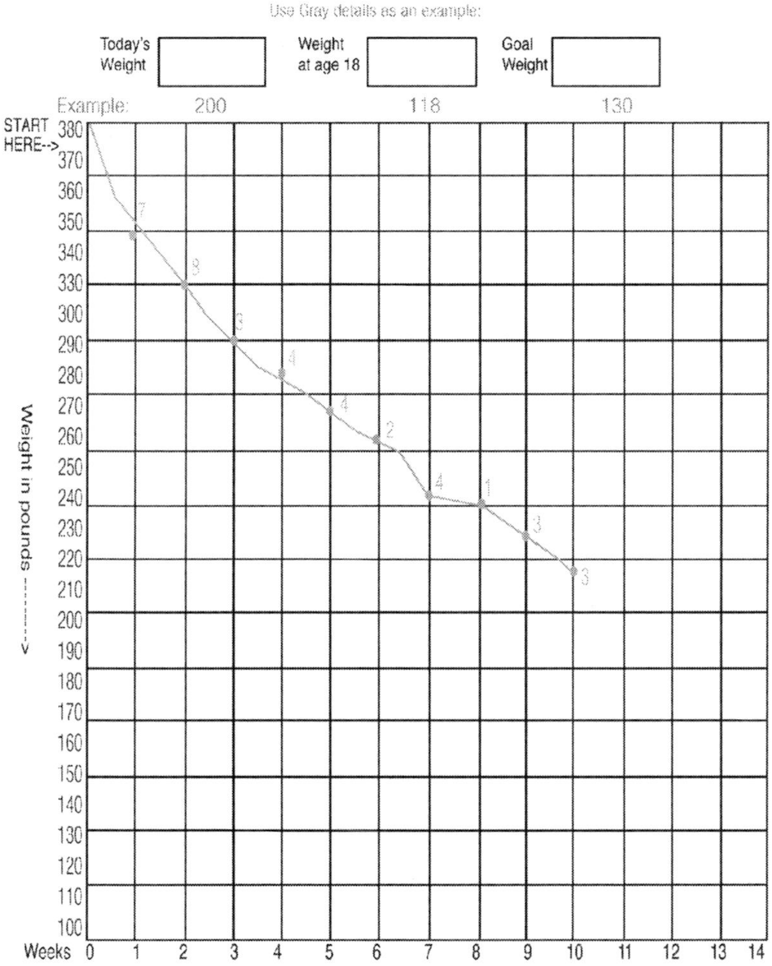

"Nothing tastes as good as thin feels"

Appendix B: Weight Chart

SmartforLife

Food Diary Log

EXCHANGE OFSFL PRODUCTS

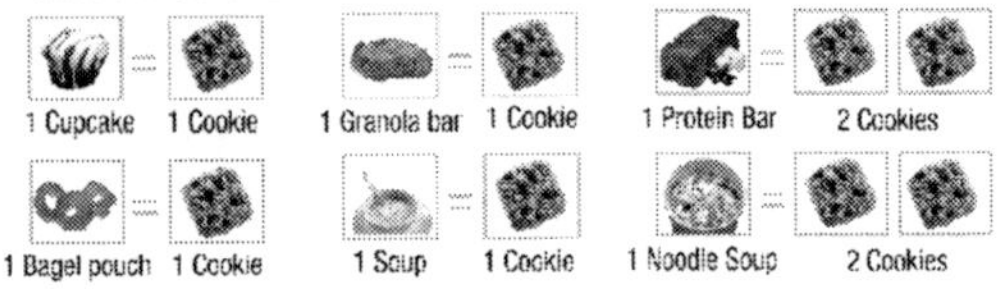

Some people do better with a food diary. Use it if you want to. Make as many copies as you need.

	EXAMPLE	MON.	TUES.	WED.	THUR.	FRI.	SAT.	SUN.
BREAKFAST	One SFL chocolate cookie with coffee.							
MIDMORNING SNACK	One SFL oatmeal cookie with water 8 oz.							
LUNCH	3 oz. of Turkey slices with salad							
MIDAFTERNOON SNACK	One SFL muffin with tea							
LATE AFTERNOON SNACK	SFL Cookie with a few almonds lots water							
DINNER	9 oz of Turkey with Kale salad							
ANYTIME SNACK	SFL shake for dessert							

Appendix C: Food Diary

SmartforLife®

My Smart Plan

	I listened to my body and ate only when hungry? (check one)	Amount of and type cardio exercise (in minutes)	Maximum Pulse Rate	Weight Training	How can I do better?
EXAMPLE	☑ Yes ☐ No If no, explain:	25 min. on treadmill & 20 min. brisk walk	148	15 ab crunches, 10 min of upper body with 5 lbs weight	Be less lazy with crunches, Do 5 more minutes on tread mill.
SUN.	☐ Yes ☐ No If no, explain:				
MON.	☐ Yes ☐ No If no, explain:				
TUE.	☐ Yes ☐ No If no, explain:				
WED.	☐ Yes ☐ No If no, explain:				
THUR.	☐ Yes ☐ No If no, explain:				
FRI.	☐ Yes ☐ No If no, explain:				
SAT.	☐ Yes ☐ No If no, explain:				

Please use this exercise planner as needed. Make as many copies as you need.

Don't forget! If you are not exercising when you start the program, don't start until you are closer to your goal. Start slow and built up slowly.

Appendix D: Exercise Planner

SmartforLife®

Meal Planner

EXCHANGE OFSFL PRODUCTS

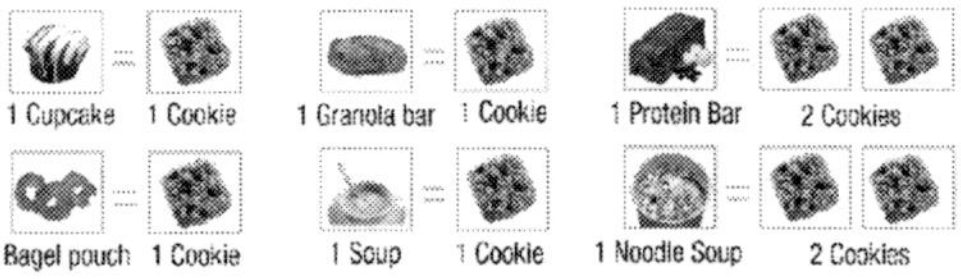

Most people do much better with their weight loss program if they plan meals a whole week ahead of time.

	MON.	TUES.	WED.	THUR.	FRI.	SAT.	SUN.
BREAKFAST							
MIDMORNING SNACK							
LUNCH							
MIDAFTERNOON SNACK							
LATE AFTERNOON SNACK							
DINNER							
ANYTIME SNACK							

Appendix E: Menu Planner

Appendix F: Website Code Where to buy Ingredients

Don't worry: you are not alone on the Smart for Life weight loss program. If you need support, or whenever you have any questions, please contact us. We would be happy to help you.

Here is the access code to the landing page of the Smart for Life website. Visit us here to look for products, recipes and information on the program or if you would like to work with us over the Internet:

Access code: www.smartforlife.com/DrSassBook

Appendix G: Live Chat with Dr. Sass

If you would like to chat online with Dr. Sass, he is available live on our website. Visit: www.smartforlife.com/DrSassBook to see what times he is available. You can talk with him online in real time about the Smart for Life program, your own diet issues, the latest science or news in the field of nutrition, and other pertinent topics.

Where to buy Smart for Life meal replacement products:
www.smartforlife.com

Where to buy Smart for Life cookie mixes:
www.smartforlife.com/DrSassBook

If you want to open a Smart For Life Center, contact us at:
Info@Smartforlife.com

If you would like to become a Smart for Life coach, email Dr. Sass at:
Drsass@smartforlife.com.

Where to buy HungerBlock: www.smartforlife.com/DrSassBook

CALIFORNIA
(888) 862-THIN

Beverly Hills
352 S. La Cienega Blvd.
Los Angeles, CA 90048
(T) 310-623-1999 (F) 310-623-1889
Center Manager: Lori Merrit
beverlyhills1@smartforlife.com

Torrance
22330 Hawthorne Boulevard, Unit D
Torrance, CA 90505
(T) 310-378-7171 (F) 310-378-7555
Center Manager: Lori Merrit
torrance1@smartforlife.com

Westlake
2772 Townsgate Road
Westlake Village, CA 91361
(T) 805-367-8440 (F) 805-367-8441
Center Manager: Kathi Mangel
westlake1@smartforlife.com

FLORIDA
(877) 701-SASS

Aventura
2980 Aventura Boulevard
Aventura, FL 33180
(T) 305-935-5550 (F) 305-935-3350
Center Manager: Gina Savage
aventura@smartforlife.com

Boca Raton
190 Glades Road, Suite E
Boca Raton, FL 33432
(T) 561-338-3999 (F) 561-338-4944
Center Manager: Renata Moulavi
bocaraton@smartforlife.com

Jupiter
2532 W. Indiantown Road, Suite A4
Jupiter, FL 33458
(T) 561-745-4888 (F) 561-745-6678
Center Manager: Nancy Greene Corn
jupiter@smartforlife.com

Orlando
451 North Maitland Avenue, Suite A
Maitland, FL 32751
(T) 407-740-0036 (F) 407-740-6091
Center Manager: Vicki Corsino
maitland@smartforlife.com

Port St. Lucie
7552 S. US 1
Port St. Lucie, FL 34952
(T) 772-293-0022 (F) 772-293-0023
Center Manager: Emily Adkins
portstlucie@smartforlife.com

South Miami
7800 SW 87th Avenue
Suite B250
Miami, FL 33173
(T) 305-270-0576 (F) 305-270-9496
Center Manager: Myra Montes de Oca
southmiami@smartforlife.com

Wellington (Royal Palm Beach)
11903 Southern Boulevard, Suite 108
Royal Palm Beach, FL 33411
(T) 561-792-2000 (F) 561-792-2090
Center Manager: Shannon Weeks
wellington@smartforlife.com

Jensen Beach
Smart for Life Med-Esthetic
Group, LLC
4239-4243 NW Federal Highway 1
Jensen Beach, FL 34957
(T) 772-692-5224
Center Manager: Emily Adkins

KANSAS

Overland Park
7960 West 135th Street, Suite 201
Overland Park, KS 66223
(T) 913-825-4333 (F) 913-825-4340
Center Manager: Debbie Dietz
overlandpark@smartforlife.com

Wichita
6611 E Central Ave., Suite B
Wichita, KS 67206
(T) 316.295.2900 (F) 316.295.2902
Center Manager: Michelle Davidson
wichita@smartforlife.com

NEW JERSEY

(866) THIN-230
Cherry Hill, New Jersey
1907 Greentree Road
Cherry Hill, NJ 08003
(T) 856-424-4747 (F) 856-424-1981
Center Manager: Beverly Parkinson

NEW YORK

(866) 410-5175
Westbury (Long Island)
1065 Old Country Road, Suite 209
Westbury, NY 11590
(T) 516-385-6225 (F) 516-385-6218
Center Manager: Amy Britt
westbury@smartforlife.com

PENNSYLVANIA

(866) THIN-230

King of Prussia
234 Mall Boulevard, Suite 150
King of Prussia, PA 19406-2954
(T) 610-265-6780 (F) 610-265-6782
Center Manager: Jonetta Carroll
kingofprussia@smartforlife.com

Langhorne
680 Middletown Blvd, Ste 100
Langhorne, PA 19047
(T) 215-752-2211 (F) 215-359-6275
Center Manager: Beverly Parkinson
langhorne@smartforlife.com

TEXAS

22698 Professional Drive
Suite 100B
Kingwood, TX 77229
(T) 281-358-5574 (F) 281-358-9677
Center Manager: Kami White
kingwood@smartforlife.com

CANADA

Montreal
6525 Boulevard Decarie, GR3
Montreal, Quebec H3W 3E3
(T) 514-489-8840 (F) 514-489-1668
Center Manager: Shoula Moulavi
montreal@smartforlife.com

How to find a Smart for Life Weight Management Center near you:

Dr. Sass sees patients at the Smart for Life Weight Management Center, 190 Glades Road, Suite E, Boca Raton, Florida 33432 (561.338.3999); for other locations in the US and Canada, look on our website: www.smartforlife.com.

About the Author

Sasson Moulavi, M.D., is the Medical Director of Smart for Life Weight Management Centers headquartered in Boca Raton, Florida. Dr. Sass is a graduate of the University of Toronto where he received the degree of Doctor of Medicine. He completed his postgraduate training at McGill University in Montreal. He holds Board Certification in Bariatric Medicine and is a member of the American Society of Bariatric Physicians. He has completed the Annual Practical Approaches to the Treatment of Obesity at Harvard University and is a member of the American Board of Anti-Aging Medicine as well as the American Academy of Anti-Aging Medicine.

It was while practicing emergency room medicine in Canada that Dr. Sass began to notice the link between being overweight and ill health and chronic disease in an increasingly younger patient population. He observed the toll excess weight was taking on his patients' lives. When a young family man died from premature heart disease on Dr. Sass's watch, he decided to dedicate his life to helping his overweight patients.

For more than 13 years, Dr. Sass has specialized in the study and treatment of bariatric medicine. He has directed the operation of multiple weight loss centers in both the United States and Canada. His hugely successful company, Smart for Life, has dozens of physician-supervised weight loss centers, a popular interactive website, and a line of natural, organic, hunger-suppressing foods and beverages. Because Dr. Sass is passionate about protecting our planet, he advocates the adoption of a natural, mostly organic diet and encourages parents, consumers, and the food industry to provide healthy, environmentally sound food choices for generations to come.

Dr. Sass lives in Boca Raton, Florida, with his wife and family.

CPSIA information can be obtained at www.ICGtesting.com
Printed in the USA
LVOW041740190212

269381LV00003B/1/P

9 781934 209929